Weight Loss

Shred Body Fat

Written By James Chappel

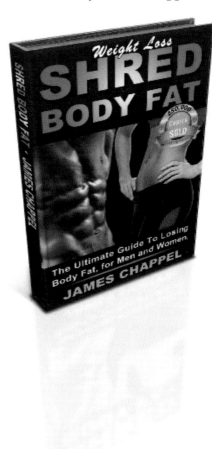

Disclaimer

Introduction

CONGRATULATIONS on purchasing this book. I am confident that within the following pages, you will discover and learn the correct way to remove stored fat from your body. This book is suitable for anyone who desires to lose real weight in the form of body fat. I will be providing you with safe, practical methods for shredding fat, as well as the proper nutrition required to work in harmony with your body. This means you will be burning fat in a completely natural way. It will not involve extreme dieting or ridiculous exercise programs, but it will involve planning, balance and discipline.

In the United States of America, over 50% of people are overweight. This means that less than half of the population carries a healthy amount of body fat. At some stage, this excess fat storage will create health problems   in the lives of the people carrying it. It is scary to think that so many people put their lives in danger, purely by neglecting their bodies and their weight. For health reasons alone, shredding body fat is a wise investment for you, your future and your family. Sculpting and achieving the lean, fit body that you want, simply becomes an added bonus and reward for your success.

Shred Body Fat will provide you with the best practical method for transforming the way that your body operates, without disrupting your lifestyle. My goal is to show you the exact process for losing as much stored body fat as you desire. I also want to give you a smooth reading experience, so that you can get straight to business. This means you will not find information that is not directly related to shredding body fat. None of the information here is theory. It is all scientifically proven to work. This book is simply a guide for you to study, learn and achieve a lean, shredded body, as soon as possible.

This book is not about goal setting, it is about getting definite results. You won't find a bunch of inspirational quotes and affirmations. If you want that, go to a Tony Robbins seminar. What you will find though, is a compact, precise tool to facilitate your desire to have the body that you envision as perfect for you. In front of you, is possibly the best and most accurate information ever written on how to lose body fat. What you take from it and how you use it, is entirely up to you. The process of shredding body fat is certainly no mystery. It is actually quite simple, provided you do the correct things and have a little patience. Just like many miracles in in life which are simplistic by nature, so is *Shred Body Fat*.

Obesity Problems

A person reaches the point of obesity when their body has reached a certain percentage of body fat. For men it is over 25% and for women it is over 32%. These are just general numbers, but anywhere near these figures can mean that many health risks become a concern. The more overweight a person is, the more risk they are placed at.

The health problems connected to obesity are:

- High blood pressure

- Heart disease and stroke

- Diabetes

- Cancer

- Gallbladder disease and gallstones.

- Asthma

- Osteoarthritis

- Gout

I have no intention of scaring you with the negative contingencies associated with obesity. My job is to keep you well clear of them and help you to design the strong, fit and healthy body that you want. Most people are not obese, but wouldn't mind losing a few pounds. Others are close to being obese and in need of help. The people who actually are obese, must use *Shred Body Fat* to completely turn their life around. Whatever point you are at, you can use this book to understand fat and shred it quickly.

Common Myths and Facts

✘ Myth – Certain foods burn fat.

✓ Fact – Currently there is no scientific evidence to prove that any type of food or supplement can burn fat directly. Foods that are high in fiber may create a feeling of fullness after a meal and require the body to burn more energy during digestion, than other foods. Those high-fiber foods can be considered a smarter choice to eat.

✗ Myth – Carbohydrates turn to fat in humans.

✓ Fact – Carbohydrates are a primary source of energy for muscles and the human brain. Humans do not carry the enzymes to convert carbohydrate into fat. The process is explained further into this book.

✗ Myth – All calories are equal.

✓ Fact – Calories that you consume from various macronutrients (carbohydrate, protein, fat) perform different functions in the body. Therefore, comparing units of energy in protein and carbohydrate, is like comparing a car to a house. They provide different services. All calories are measured in the same units of energy (calories or kilojoules) so that they have some level of congruence, but in reality, they cannot be compared.

✗ Myth – There is no one perfect way to lose weight.

✓ Fact – It stands true that everyone is different, but the science of losing body fat remains the same for everyone. The rate or speed that fat-loss occurs in different people may vary, but when the correct principles are applied, anyone can achieve their desired weight.

✖ Myth – If you stop working out, your muscle will turn into fat.

✓ Fact – Muscle cannot turn into fat. They are two different things. When you stop working out, you lose the muscle that you previously gained. This can make you less firm and more flabby, which can make you feel like you have gained body fat.

✖ Myth – Weight training will make you look like a bodybuilder.

✓ Fact – Weight training or resistance training will slightly tear muscle. This will enable you to rebuild it, but the result will not make you look like a bodybuilder. In fact, not even close. It is impossible for anyone to look much bigger just by training with weights. Lifting weights will simply make your muscles stronger and more dense, thus creating another fat-burning tool for your body to use.

✖ Myth – You get all the vitamins that you need from food.

✓ Fact – Most people do not even come close to acquiring sufficient vitamins from their diet. This can result in energy loss, fatigue, a weak immune system and recurring sickness. Fixing this can be as simple as taking a multivitamin with breakfast each day.

✖ Myth – Diets are difficult.

✓ Fact – Deprivation is difficult, diets are not. Once you remove the deprivation of food in a diet, it then becomes a meal plan. A meal plan does not consist of food cravings or boredom. A meal plan simply provides your body and brain with sufficient energy to get through the day, without the feeling of being deprived.

✖ Myth – Cellulite is a skin condition.

✓ Fact – Cellulite is an appearance by the skin, as a result of stored body fat. In this case, the fat has left the body's fat cells and is trapped by connective tissue. Removing cellulite is as simple as shredding unwanted fat in that particular area of the body.

✖ Myth – Eating too much sugar causes diabetes.

✓ Fact – Diabetes is not caused by simply eating too much sugar. Type 1 diabetes is hereditary, while Type 2 diabetes is caused by an unhealthy lifestyle and obesity.

✖ Myth – A fat-free diet requires cutting all fats from your diet.

✓ Fact – A fat-free diet requires cutting all non-essential fats from your diet, but still consuming "good" fats. These fats are essential to your health and can assist you in losing stored body fat.

1. Knowledge of Food

Carbohydrate

Foods containing carbohydrate are essential for good health. They are your body and your brain's main source of fuel, while also providing important vitamins, minerals, antioxidants and fiber. These are all necessary for your body to function in a healthy manner and avoid problems such as heart disease, diabetes, hypertension, constipation, and many other diseases.

Carbohydrates consist of sugar, fruit, vegetables, wheat, rice, pasta, cereals, grains, starches, legumes and any other food which is not a protein or a fat. They form the majority of the foods that we eat in a normal, balanced diet. Certain foods are made up of both carbohydrate and protein, such as beans, milk and nuts. These carbohydrates tend to be digested slower and they usually contain more nutrients than empty carbohydrates, such as table sugar. Despite this being the case, ALL carbohydrates will be broken down easily, to be used by the body as a preferred source of energy.

Protein

In simple terms, protein is made up of long chains of amino acids. Amino acids are biochemical molecules containing carbon, hydrogen, oxygen and nitrogen. These combine into different structures to form the various types of protein within the body. There are 22 amino acids which are essential and are required by the body for proper functioning.

After we eat food, protein is broken down during digestion and separated into individual amino acids. These amino acids are then absorbed and reformed to make new proteins, which are used by the body. The 22 types of amino acids are divided into two groups: essential and non-essential amino acids. There are 8 essential and 14 non-essential amino acids. Non-essential amino acids can be created by the body, but essential amino acids can only be obtained from food.

There are many forms of protein, which all play an important role in body functioning. For example, collagen is a protein and is vital for the strength, elasticity and composition of our hair, nails and skin. The amino acids in protein are also responsible for enzymes, hormones, immune system antibodies, as well as the growth or repair of bone and muscle tissue. Sources of protein include chicken, turkey, red meat, ham, fish, eggs, milk, whey, cheese, beans, nuts, legumes and certain vegetables.

IMPORTANT ⇒ **The body can only use so much protein in a single meal.**

This is something that many personal trainers, athletes and even some nutrition experts do not know. There is absolutely no value in consuming excess protein. Eating too much protein puts a tremendous strain on the kidneys, until the body eventually urinates it out. Ultimately, eating too much protein will NOT build more muscle and will simply go to waste.

Fat

There are basically 2 types of fat in our daily lives. The fat we consume in food, and the fat that sits around our waist and belly area. I'm sure that most people have been able to identify with the latter at some stage in life. The body is programmed to store body fat very easily, in case we somehow happen to run out of food. It is a survival mechanism of the human anatomy. This stored body fat also provides you with energy in between meals, until you are able to feed your body with the next meal. For these reasons, stored body fat serves its purpose. The fat that we eat in our food can come in different forms. It is usually found in the form of an oily substance (olive oil, canola oil, soybean oil, etc) or the form of a solid fat (butter, margarine, bacon fat, etc). Fats are usually hidden in our foods. Therefore, without looking at the nutritional facts or ingredients, there is no way of knowing that they are there.

The fat that is in any meal we eat, has a destiny once digested. Its destiny is NOT to be used a fuel straight after we eat. Its destiny is to travel from the intestines, through the bloodstream, and to be stored around the body in fat cells. When the body has finished using the carbohydrate (in a meal) as its primary source of energy, insulin is cleared and fat is retrieved for energy use. Only then, will fat be used by muscles in the body and burnt as fuel.

Lipoprotein is a form of cholesterol which the body produces naturally, and is responsible for transporting fats to different areas of the body. This fat can be used by the liver, used as slow muscle fuel, or simply stored. LDL (low-density lipoprotein) is the "bad" cholesterol that is responsible for taking fat and storing it around your body in places such as your arteries. HDL (high-density lipoprotein) is the "good" cholesterol that is responsible for removing stored cholesterol in arteries, and transporting it to the liver. Fat within the liver is broken down to form hormones, while cholesterol is broken down into bile. This bile dissolves fat, making it digestible for enzymes produced by the pancreas and intestinal lining.

The human body uses "good" fats (essential fatty acids) in food to carry out tasks and to keep the body functioning in a healthy manner. The other fats in food are either used as a source of energy throughout the day, or stored as body fat. On a regular day of balanced eating, the average woman will burn a minimum 40 grams of body fat per day, and the average man will burn a minimum 60 grams per day. These numbers represent what is required from fat, as a secondary source of energy during a normal day. Even when you are asleep, there are internal operations being run continuously just to keep you alive. Women and men can burn even more fat on a daily basis by being active and incorporating exercise into their day. For now though, we will look at the minimum fat required by the body every day.

The numbers, 40 (for women) and 60 (for men), can be used to calculate approximately how many grams of body fat you can expect to burn in a day, while simply eating a low-fat diet. Take a look at the table below. (*NOTE: good fats are not included in fat consumption. They are used by the body for other purposes.*)

Fat averages for a 24-hour day

Fat intake/usage (+/-)	Women (grams)	Men (grams)
Food consumed	+20g	+25g
Morning Cardio	-15g	-20g
Daily activity	-40g	-60g

Total Fat gain/loss	-35g	-55g

These numbers may not seem too impressive, but keep in mind that they are for real body fat. If you multiply these by the number of days in a month (30), you have 1050 grams of fat-loss for women! and 1650 grams of fat-loss for men! Granted, most people will not be doing cardio every single morning, but you can see that it doesn't take long to remove a big chunk of real fat from your body. The option to do so is yours.

Excess body fat is usually stored across your entire body evenly. This is the reason you may have previously lost body fat, but not noticed any change. Your belly probably looked exactly the same, so you were not made aware that you actually burnt 100 grams of fat in your upper back, arms or legs, during that week. Shredding body fat is an art. The good news is that unlike other skills which take years to master, shredding fat can be understood and achieved relatively quickly. By understanding how and why fat is stored, you have a great start.

As you continue through this book, you will find information that is vital for correctly losing body fat. These are the smart ways to burn fat directly, as well as indirectly. Once you know these, losing weight will no longer be a mystery. It will actually make complete sense. You may notice emphasis on those particular points, because I want you to finish this book being able to say, "I get it!" Think of your fat cells as a collection that you have built up gradually throughout your life. Just like, saving money in the bank. Although now, it's time to spend that money! By applying simple strategies, you will begin to shrink your "fat bank," one gram at a time.

Essential Fats

There are certain fats that are essential for our health and well-being, enabling our body to function perfectly. The body cannot produce these essential fatty acids, so they must be acquired from the food we eat. Foods that have monounsaturated and polyunsaturated fats are responsible for providing us with the essential fatty acids that our body needs. The two essential fatty acids are Omega-3 and Omega-6

Essential Fatty Acids
Omega-3 - (Alpha Linolenic Acid)
Omega-6 - (Linoleic Acid)

Good fats can be found in many foods naturally. Mono-unsaturated fats can lower bad cholesterol (LDL), and can be found in foods such as grains, nuts, avocado, olive oil and canola oil. Polyunsaturated fats contain the essential fatty acids, omega-3 and omega-6. Omega-6 can be found in safflower, sunflower and corn oils; while Omega-3 is best obtained from flaxseed oil, salmon and other oily fish. By including these good fats in your diet, you can increase your fat-loss by encouraging your body to perform at its best.

The *Shred Body Fat* program does not completely restrict you from essential fatty acids. These fats serve a purpose, which is to better your well-being and promote a healthy functioning body. Carbohydrates are used as fuel during daily activities, but omega-3 and omega-6 fatty acids are required for your body to operate perfectly. Infants require omega-3 for brain development, while adults rely on both omega-3 and omega-6 for their central nervous system and normal brain functioning. Think of it as WD-40 for the brain and nerves inside you. These essential fatty acids are not used as a source of energy, but they are used to support metabolism. They also lower blood cholesterol and guard against heart problems such as Heart Arrhythmia (irregular heartbeat).

Too Much of a Good Thing

Many people are aware of good fats and they use that as an excuse to overeat on foods that contain them. Unfortunately, once the human body has attained its daily intake of essential fats, any extra will be stored as body fat. Therefore, overeating on salmon or munching on nuts constantly throughout the day (just because they contain good fats) is not a good idea. This will equate to body fat storage. Certain oily fish also contain small amounts of saturated fat, which would be stored directly.

15

There is no recommended intake of essential fatty acids, but it is estimated that between 12-17 grams per day is adequate. It is not uncommon for me to come across a person who complains about sudden weight gain, but who also openly admits to eating a lot of salmon, avocado or nuts. The message here is clear. Eat good fats. but be careful! Eat salmon if you enjoy it, but stick to controlled portions and control how often you eat it. Eat avocado if you enjoy it, but use it lightly as a spread; do not eat it in large chunks like eating pieces of an apple. Eat nuts as a tasty treat on occasion, but do not mindlessly munch on them non-stop throughout the day. By controlling these foods, you will be getting a sufficient amount of good fats in your diet, without storing an excess. You don't want to interfere with your fat-loss goal by overeating on good fats.

Fat in Food

The fat that is found in the food we eat is split up into 3 basic categories. These are: monounsaturated, polyunsaturated, and saturated. There is also a fourth category called trans fats, which heads the list of bad fats. Trans fats are made from vegetable oils which have had hydrogen added to them. This turns a regular fat (liquid) into a more solid state. Companies use trans fats to extend the shelf life of food which they produce. Thus, making them more profitable over a longer period of time. Trans fats are mainly found in commercial products which are baked or fried. They can be seen in the list of ingredients on the packaging, but usually come in a couple of disguises. This disguises include: "partially hydrogenated oil" and "vegetable shortening." Hydrogenated oils and shortenings are fats that are responsible for clogging the internal walls of your arteries. Anything similar to the descriptions that I have mentioned above, should warn and prevent you from buying that product.

Avoid trans fats at all costs.

Saturated fats are the next worst in line. These fats are also responsible for blocking your arteries and raising your blood cholesterol. They increase LDL and decrease HDL in the bloodstream, which raises your risk of heart disease. Often, they are the last and most difficult to remove from the fat cell. They are more common than trans fats, because they appear naturally in many animal products. Small amounts of saturated fat that are found in lean meats cannot be avoided. These are minimal, but larger amounts in products can be avoided by reading the nutritional label and ingredients which are listed. When eating out at restaurants, ask your waiter what oil they are using to cook the meal that you are ordering.

On the next page, there is a list of the different types of fats and the foods that contain them. You can still eat some of the foods listed, if you choose, but be aware of the ones with "bad" fat content. At the very least, limit those particular foods and replace them with healthier options, e.g. non-fat milk instead of regular milk. As you gain experience in food selection, recognizing bad fats will become easier.

Mono-unsaturated	Poly-unsaturated	Saturated	Trans Fats
canola oil	flaxseed oil	full-cream milk	shelf donuts/cakes
olive oil	salmon/oily fish	cheese, butter	shelf muffins/pastries
nuts	sunflower oil	beef, sausages, bacon	confectionery
avocado	safflower oil	coconut oil/palm oil	snack chips/cookies

Warning: Do not expose flaxseed oil to high temperatures or cook with it (frying, baking, etc). This exposure to extreme heat, destroys the "good" fats within, turning them into "bad" fats.

De Novo Lipogenesis

The process of carbohydrate being converted into fat is called De Novo Lipogenesis. For years, scientists have conducted experiments on humans and animals, recording the effect that carbohydrate has as a source of energy and how it is stored. In every case, the outcome is different according to the species tested, but consistent within their own. Certain animals carry specific enzymes which convert carbohydrate and store it as fat. A perfect example is a cow. Cows are large animals that expend a lot of energy (calories) throughout the day, by slowly moving around, but they only eat a limited amount of food. This food is carbohydrate in the form of grass. Their body composition allows them to eat carbohydrate throughout the day and store it as fat, despite eating very little. Pigs are also able to easily fatten themselves on a diet of grains, throughout the day. These farm animals DO carry the enzymes necessary to convert carbohydrate easily and store it as fat. Their diet consists almost entirely of carbohydrates in the form of wheat, grains, and grass, while consistently storing it in the form of adipose tissue (fat), for later use.

The human body operates in a completely different way. In fact, it carries an entirely different set of enzymes that do not promote De Novo Lipogenesis. The enzymes within the human body are programmed strictly to convert carbohydrate into glycogen and use it as a primary source of energy. Carbohydrate is stored as glycogen in the liver, while the pancreas produces insulin. This insulin distributes any extra glycogen to muscles around the body. Carbohydrate is NOT converted into fat.

Even large amounts of carbohydrate intake will be used as energy and will not be stored as fat. The average human body is capable of storing more than 500g of carbohydrates at a single time. Unused carbohydrate will be stored as glycogen in the muscles of the body, until it is eventually used as energy or oxidized hours later through body heat. The human body is simply programmed to use carbohydrate as immediate energy, unlike our farm animal friends. It is fair to say that the more carbohydrate you eat, the more you will burn. There has been countless scientific studies that have proved this beyond doubt.

A case experiment consisting of a human drinking 5 litres of Coco-Cola in one sitting had resulted in no fat storage. As you can imagine, this is an overdose of pure sugar in the form of soda, yet it resulted in zero fat gain. Another case study had groups of people consume the equivalent of 500g of carbohydrate in a single sitting. The people tested were consuming carbohydrate in the form of bread, rice, and other starches. Despite this huge carbohydrate intake, zero fat storage was again recorded through De Novo Lipogenesis. Five hundred grams of carbohydrate is more food than most people would eat in an entire day, let alone one single meal! This was was certainly a case of extreme overeating.

I can give you many examples of official scientific case studies and research proving De Novo Lipogenesis to be of little occurrence in humans, but that is not what this book is about. This book is about getting you on the right track towards shredding body fat, as soon as possible. Nobody with the intent to lose weight is concerned with eating ridiculous amounts of carbohydrate, but understanding the process of De Novo Lipogenesis in humans is essential to reaching your fat-loss goal. The sooner you realize that sugars, starches, and all forms of carbohydrate have very little chance of turning into fat, within your body, the sooner you will reach your fat-loss goal. I am not saying that you should overeat and splurge on carbohydrates, just because they will not be converted into fat. What I am saying is that you should not think of carbohydrate as your enemy. Unfortunately many people do, and this destroys their chances of losing real body fat.

Carbohydrates are your friend. The entire *Shred Body Fat* program is designed so that you can use carbohydrates efficiently, in a way that boosts your metabolism and promotes fat-loss. If you are still not convinced or are skeptical about carbohydrate and its unlikelihood of being converted into fat (in humans), *Google.com* has countless books on the subject. Just go to *Google Books* and search for *De Novo Lipogenesis*. There, you will find all the scientific evidence that you will ever need, for free.

Carbohydrate – In more detail...

Now that I've explained the scientific term of *De Novo Lipogenesis*, it's time to take a closer look at carbohydrate itself. As we now know, carbohydrate or sugar does NOT get converted into body fat (unless you're a cow). A lot of so-called professionals are hesitant to recommend a carbohydrate enriched diet. This makes people think that a diet which is high in carbohydrate, is a bad thing. There is all sorts of confusion and ignorance associated with carbohydrate and its role within the body.

What is the function of carbohydrate?

Carbohydrate is a macronutrient that is essential to the human body. Not only is it essential, but it plays the role of the body's primary source of energy and is the only source of fuel that your brain can use. Without it, your brain simply cannot function properly. Any time you are deprived of carbohydrate, even when replacing it with protein or fat in your diet, you are temporarily starving your body and your brain. This is the reason why people on low carbohydrate diets can become easily irritable. Their healthy level of serotonin (which the body produces naturally when eating carbohydrate) becomes disrupted. With time, it can lead to more serious mood declines or depression. We all know the temperamental feelings or mood swings that occur when we are hungry and haven't eaten for a long period of time. This is the exact same thing that happens when the body is deprived of carbohydrate. Concentration becomes affected, and you are prone to making mistakes in everyday life.

21

The digestion of carbohydrate is a relatively speedy process. It becomes available as a source of energy almost immediately. After a meal is eaten, protein and fat are separated; while the intestines go straight to work, by converting carbohydrate into glycogen. Different types of carbohydrate are actually the same, in the sense that they are all absorbed and transformed into glycogen. Once carbohydrate has become glycogen, it can then be stored. As mentioned previously, some glycogen is stored in the liver to be used as energy by the body immediately. The remainder of the glycogen is sent out and stored in muscles for further use. Now that you know the human body can store large amounts of carbohydrate at any one time (over 500 grams), you should also be made aware that the process of storing carbohydrate is completely natural.

Anytime you feel extremely hungry, the first thing that you should do is eat some sort of carbohydrate. Even candy would be sufficient, because your body and brain is sending you a signal to eat! Cutting carbs in any way, shape or form, is a type of starvation. Your body will respond to this by slowing down, while your concentration and physical performance will also become affected. These signs are the direct result of removing or limiting carbohydrate in your diet.

Insulin

When you eat and digest food, the pancreas releases a hormone called insulin. This hormone allows the cells of the body to absorb food and energy in the form of glycogen. The glycogen is then used as energy by your body in daily life. Think of insulin like a drill that creates holes in cells, which enables glucose to enter easily. It's a natural process which is essential in contributing to healthy functioning of the body. Insulin is also responsible for transporting amino acids to cells in the body, as well as delivering glycogen to the brain. Essentially, insulin is like an umbilical cord for the brain, which delivers energy 24 hours a day.

Insulin is always present in tiny amounts throughout the bloodstream. When the amount of insulin increases, after a meal, fat storage can occur easily. This is because insulin activates or inhibits various enzymes that are responsible for removing fat from its storage cell (fat cell). As a result, the body programs itself to store the fat that you consume in a meal, while it uses carbohydrate as fuel. Once the insulin has finished doing its job and has almost totally cleared, the body can then prepare itself to release fat from fat cells. This is the time that fat can be used as energy. This entire process may take 2-3 hours, depending on the size of your meal.

Unfortunately, many so-called experts take this natural process and use it to manipulate weight-loss. Their theory is that once you prevent insulin from occurring, you can use fat as a primary source of energy. They achieve this by using a low-carbohydrate diet, which consists of a high percentage of protein or fat. Not only is this an unreliable weight-loss strategy, but it can also subtract from your muscle-mass and your overall health. One other thing that low-carb advocates either forget to tell you or simply do not know, is that protein also produces insulin.

Tests have been done by some of the world's leading bioscientists, which measure insulin levels after protein consumption. In some cases, the insulin released for protein is even greater than for carbohydrate. Below, is a graph which clearly illustrates the amounts of insulin released into the bloodstream after various carbohydrate or protein consumption.

INSULIN RELEASED INTO BLOODSTREAM

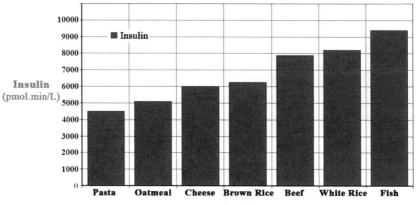

Foods
(Carbohydrate and Protein)

As you see, fish and beef produce substantially higher amounts of insulin than pasta and brown rice. Even cheese with its high fat content, still produces higher results than pasta or oatmeal. White rice is the highest of the carbohydrates to produce an insulin release, but still outdone by fish and only just ahead of beef. This study proves that insulin serves many other purposes besides storing carbohydrate.

What about Atkins?

Robert Atkins was a cardiologist whose first book came out in the early 70's and continued to have success for more than 30 years. His diet is commonly known as "The Atkins Diet" and it was well promoted as a wonder discovery. Atkins's book sold millions of copies based on ketosis. Ketosis is a process that the body goes through when carbohydrates are almost completely removed from a diet. The Atkins Diet allows for any type of protein or fat to be consumed in replacement for carbohydrate. Protein and fat in the body then become a primary source of energy due to an insulin delay and absence of carbohydrate. There is also no emphasis on

24

controlling calorie intake, provided carbohydrate intake is almost zero.

In years to come, the Atkins Diet became the quintessential "fad diet." The reason this diet became so popular and is still used even until this day, is because it tricks people into thinking that they have lost weight. They look leaner, feel leaner and become convinced that their diet is working. In reality, their weight-loss is almost entirely water and muscle weight. A bad result. The minute their normal diet resumes, the body comes out of ketosis and all the lost weight is returned. Ketosis is an unhealthy loophole in achieving weight-loss. It serves no purpose towards real fat-loss, while depriving the body of essential nutrients.

As stated previously, modern-day research proves that many proteins produce an even higher release of insulin into the bloodstream than certain carbohydrates. For example, beef produces more insulin than pasta or brown rice, while fish releases more insulin than white rice. Your body releases insulin naturally for both carbohydrate and protein in a meal, and this process should not be disturbed or altered. In fact, excess ketone bodies that are produced from ketosis, can make blood more acidic. This deprives cells in the body of oxygen. When cells do not have oxygen, they will eventually die.

Ketosis also presents some obvious side effects such as bad breath, dehydration, mood swings and headaches. People persist through these, because they like the results that they see from their diet. Who wouldn't? A few minor problems seem fine when you've dropped 10-20 pounds in weight! Unfortunately, the joy that comes from losing so much weight is always short lived. Some people do try to prolong the return of their lost weight by continuing to put their body under this type of strain. Inevitably, their failure becomes clear once they resume a normal diet, and stop treating themselves like a science experiment.

Atkins encouraged his readers to persist with the diet so that they kept the weight off, but he never mentioned the long-term health risks associated with consuming high amounts of fat and protein. Heart disease, high cholesterol, high blood pressure, kidney failure, malnutrition; just to name a few. Any time your body goes into ketosis, you have taken two steps backwards. Ketosis delays your potential to lose real body fat by shifting your metabolism and sending it in the complete opposite direction of carbohydrate and the purpose it serves. Whether Atkins was aware of the dangers involved by using his diet or not, he was light-years away from helping people to shred body fat.

Diabetes

What is it?

Diabetes is a disorder of which the body cannot use carbohydrate properly. If not treated, diabetes can lead to damage in nerves and blood vessels. Such problems can increase the risk of heart disease, stroke, and damage to other major organs of the body. Without going into too much detail about diabetes (as this book is about fat-loss, not diabetes), I will explain the different types.

1) Type 1 Diabetes is more often considered hereditary. It can be found in children or young adults and it relates to the pancreas producing insufficient insulin. Monitored treatment and insulin injections are required.

2) Type 2 Diabetes is the more common type of diabetes, occurring in up to 90% of cases. It happens when the body's cells resist insulin, thus preventing glucose storage. This type of diabetes is mostly attributed to obesity and an unhealthy, inactive lifestyle. Successful treatment can be achieved by an improvement in

lifestyle, through proper diet and exercise. In some cases, pills or insulin may be required.

3) Gestational Diabetes can occur in women during pregnancy, but is usually cured after the baby is born. Women who develop this type of diabetes are placed at high risk of developing Type 2 Diabetes within years to come. Treatment is the same as for Type 2 Diabetes.

Sugar Does Not Cause Diabetes

Table sugar itself is actually compounded by part sucrose and part fructose. This gives it a lower effect on blood sugar and insulin levels than glucose and some other starches, such as potatoes, white rice and bread. So, despite containing very little nutritional value, sugar is not the evil villain that most people think it is. If you are hungry and unable to get food, it is actually a wise decision to eat something containing sugar or even high-sugar. This will suppress your hunger and feed your body, muscles and brain, until you find a more balanced meal.

There is no medical evidence to prove that sugar or carbohydrate causes diabetes. Insulin is a natural reaction to the consumption of food in general, not just carbohydrates. The more food you eat, the more insulin your body requires. Diabetes is a disease that is either hereditary or created from an unhealthy lifestyle and obesity. Sugar alone, is not responsible for diabetes. Additionally, medical research has shown that a balanced diet containing complex carbohydrates, actually improves glucose control.

Complex and Simple Carbohydrates

For many years, there has been much confusion associated with the difference between complex carbohydrates and simple carbohydrates. Some nutritionists still get these two mixed up. Complex carbohydrates are chains of three or more single sugar molecules linked together to form one food. Foods such as: pasta, rice, bread, corn, potato and fruit - all fall within the complex carbohydrate category. The important role that these foods play is their nutritional contribution to the body. Simple carbs such as: candy, sports drinks, and table sugar - all have very little nutrition. This is why they can be labeled as "empty carbs."

Foods like rice, potato, and bread have been given a bad name over the years and are wrongly placed in the simple carbs category. This is only because they can raise insulin rapidly and cause a higher spike in blood sugar (compared to other carbohydrates), when eaten alone. Depending on the type of carbohydrate consumed, insulin levels will vary. As mentioned previously in the chapter about insulin, this process is completely normal. The correct way to manage these carbohydrates is to balance them by adding a portion of protein to your meals. That way, your energy levels can be more consistent and you will still keep the goodness and nutrition which all complex carbohydrates contain.

Carbohydrates which are complex but are still converted into blood sugar relatively quickly (rice, bread, potato), should not be avoided. They should be used to supply your body with fuel, just like any other carbohydrate. The fact that they spike your insulin levels even more than an empty carbohydrate such as table sugar, does not undermine their value. By balancing your meals with protein and good fats, you can still feed your body with the essential nutrients it needs, without an insulin spike.

> **Weight control is almost entirely associated with food eaten and energy burnt, not insulin levels.**

Despite making it clear that insulin levels are not something you should be concerning yourself with, I feel that there is much to gain in becoming familiar with which carbohydrates take longer to digest and be converted into blood sugar (glycogen). Having this knowledge can help you decide which carbohydrates will keep you feeling fuller for longer. This gives you the power to create meals that contain slow releasing carbohydrates, made even slower with the addition of protein and good fats. This is something that may be beneficial before bedtime, when your metabolism is getting ready to settle for the night. Most importantly, you will gain more control over your energy levels throughout the day.

Above all, I must stress that *Shred Body Fat* starts with proper eating habits, correct exercise and a balance in lifestyle. The *Shred* diet (meal plan) encourages you to feed your body carbohydrates as a primary source of energy. This intake is then balanced by the activity that you use on a daily basis to burn it off. Therefore, expanding your knowledge of various carbohydrates and how quickly they are converted into glycogen is optional, not mandatory. It can simply help you make better decisions and teach you more about how your energy levels respond to different carbs. The next chapter contains the source for that information, if you desire to add it to your knowledge of carbohydrate. It's called, The Glycemic Index.

The Glycemic Index

The Glycemic Index is a list of all carbohydrates, which contains a rating that measures their impact on blood sugar levels. Glucose is generally found at the top of the list with a score of 102. This means that it is almost pure blood sugar, and requires very little time for conversion into glycogen. Carbohydrates that fall into the low-medium range (fruit, multi-grain bread, pasta) generally have a Glycemic Index (GI) between 30-60. These are considered smart food choices for balancing your energy levels and staying fuller for longer.

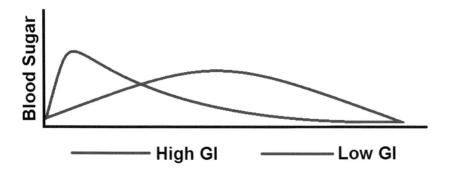

The diagram above shows the effect of two different carbohydrate foods which have the same amount of calories, but a different GI. The low GI food (blue line) clearly shows a more consistent and balanced flow of energy. Thus, producing less of a spike in blood sugar levels.

Glycemic Index relates to the type of carbohydrate in food, not how much carbohydrate is in food. The ranking system that measures the ratio of blood sugar increase, in comparison to a specific food portion (100g), is the Glycemic Load (GL). As far as losing body fat goes, there is no evidence to prove that eating low GI or low GL contributes greatly to weight- loss. This is because your body produces insulin naturally to store whatever carbohydrate you consume, whether your blood sugar is spiked or not. Despite this, the meals that you choose to eat while shredding body fat, shall always contain sensible GI levels. This is simply because you will be adding portions of protein to them. Anytime protein or fat is added to a meal, the glycemic effect of the meal as a whole, can be reduced.

Now you know that low GI carbohydrates are not absolutely necessary, they can still be a beneficial part of your diet. Low GI carbs can add even more balance to your meals and they generally tend to be quite nutritious. At the other end of the scale, many high GI foods (white rice, whole grain bread, vegetables) can also have great nutrition. Again, you can still eat these without spiking your energy levels, simply by mixing them with low GI foods or protein.

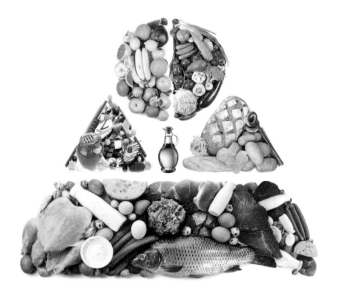

Comparing The Effects of Different Carbohydrates

Below are 3 graphs comparing the Glycemic Index

for different foods.

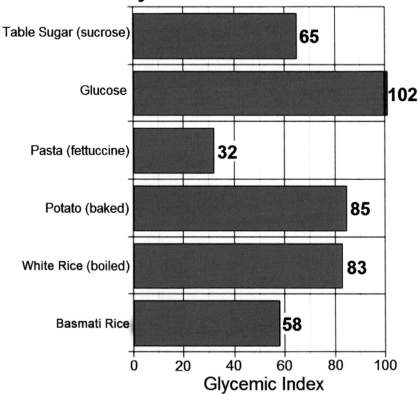

In the graph above, you can see that table sugar has a relatively high GI at 65. Glucose tops the chart at 102, and is generally what all other foods are compared to. Next on the list is pasta at a low 32. The semolina in pasta is responsible for slowing down carbohydrate conversion, making it a smart choice if eaten in controlled portions. Potato and rice both have a much higher GI at 85 and 83 respectively. Finally, basmati rice at 58. is a good alternative to white rice, in terms of lowering blood sugar spike.

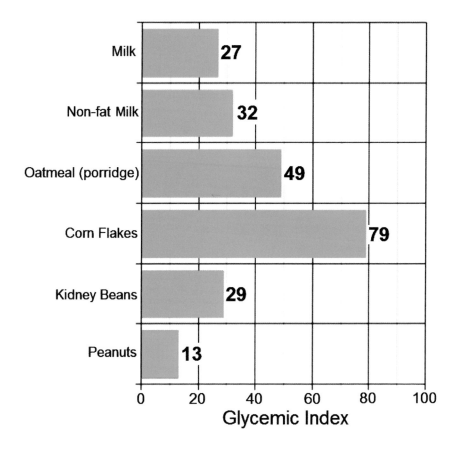

This second graph (above) starts off by showing the low GI of regular milk (27). Non-fat milk has a slightly higher GI (32), due to the absence of fat. Cow's milk, in general, is slow to digest;

hence, the low GI in all types. Next on the list, is oatmeal. It is a great choice over corn flakes, for stabilizing morning blood sugar levels. When combined with milk, GI is lowered even further. Lastly, the protein in kidney beans gives them a low GI, while peanuts have both protein and high fat (low 13).

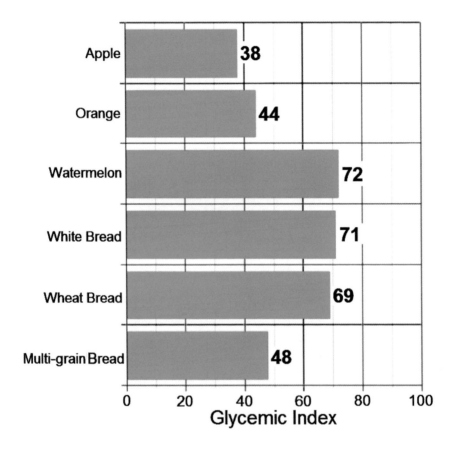

The final graph (above) shows the naturally low GI of an apple and an orange. Watermelon has a much higher GI (72), but because it contains very few calories, its effect on blood sugar is usually minimal. Next, you can see that white bread and wheat bread have very little GI difference. Despite wheat bread offering more nutrition and fiber, its conversion to blood sugar is still quite fast. Alternatively, multi-grain bread provides a lower GI (48), because it has grains that slow down digestion.

> **Note:** *Not all Glycemic Indexes are exactly the same. The GI for a particular food may vary slightly, depending on where and which country they were tested.*

Be aware that the Glycemic Index of a particular food, should be compared to the amount of calories being consumed from that food. This affects the overall impact of that food on your blood sugar levels (the Glycemic Load). A general understanding of GI and smart portion control, usually accounts for this. As you can see in the graph above, watermelon has a fairly fast rate of conversion to blood sugar (high GI) in your body; but as a food energy source, it contains very few calories. This means that you would have to eat a lot of watermelon in one meal, for it to affect your blood sugar in a major way. In most cases, foods with a high GI but few calories, would have very little impact on the overall GI of a meal.

Pasta (made from semolina) has the complete opposite effect. It has a low Glycemic Index, but is quite concentrated in calories. Therefore, after consuming pasta, you will have an abundance of energy, but it will be distributed slowly over a period of time. Incidentally, pasta has been given a bad name for many years, as a carbohydrate that is fattening. This is entirely false information. It is the extras that people add to pasta (cheese, oil, dressing, cream, etc) that make it fattening; not the pasta itself. The calories in pasta are of high nutritional value, while the semolina that it contains, lowers its GI. As a result, pasta is one of the best foods that you could eat prior to working out, or a lengthy period of time without food.

2. Tools for Shredding

Muscle

Muscle is tissue composed of fibres which expand and contract to control the way that your body moves. These movements respond to the signals that your brain delivers. Absolutely everything that you conceive of with your brain is expressed as muscular motion. It would be impossible for you to do anything without your muscles. Your muscle mass is also responsible for shredding fat and burning energy 24 hours a day. It is the storing ground for glycogen, which enables you to burn it as fuel. The more muscle that you have, the faster your Resting and Basal Metabolic Rate (RMR and BMR) will be.

For metabolic purposes, it makes sense to protect your muscle, and work towards increasing it. This can become a challenge when you are shredding body fat, which is why your gym sessions require your best effort. Even by simply maintaining your current muscle mass while lowering body fat levels, you will help keep your fat-burning engine running at its peak. As you continue to shred fat, your muscles will become more defined and noticeable. This can serve as great incentive and motivation to stay focused on your goal.

During *Shred Body Fat*, it is impossible to prevent muscle loss from occurring, simply because you will be using a slight calorie deficit to shred fat. Shredding fat is your first priority, but only to the point where you can easily rebuild muscle soon after it is lost.

Your muscle maintenance will be easier to accomplish with a continual resistance training program. Try not to miss any gym sessions. Muscle-loss can accumulate quickly when shredding fat each day, so avoid it. If you stay on top of your resistance training, it will never feel like you have to struggle to catch up on lost muscle and strength. Instead, you will always feel that you are keeping your strength while gradually shredding the unwanted fat from your body.

Does muscle turn to fat?

So many people fear that if they stop working out or training, their muscle will turn directly to fat. This is impossible. Muscle and fat are two completely different things. They cannot change from one to another any easier than concrete can change into wood. You may have noticed that if you have ever stopped working out for a period of time, there was a difference in your body shape. That difference may have felt like you had gained weight, but not so. It was simply an illusion.

The illusion that I am talking about happens as a result of a couple things. When muscles are no longer used in a way that enables them to stay strong, they lose their size, firmness and density. They can turn flabby and give the impression that they have turned to fat. Since there is so much muscle within the body, it is very easy to feel like you have gained weight from this. Another event that occurs when people stop working out, is water retention. The body is capable of holding on to extra water, which along with the loose muscle, can make you feel like you have gained 20 pounds! Again, this is just an illusion.

The good news is that it will not take long to get your toned, fit body back. Once you start training again, it can be a matter of just a few days before you regain your muscle and drop the water weight that you are carrying. In some cases, people return to the gym stronger and refreshed, because their body has fully recovered after the time off. Real weight-gain will only occur during time off, when a person or an athlete eats the same large amounts of food as when they were training.

The Hunger Signal

The key to shredding body fat is your metabolism. The way that you influence your metabolism is what will determine your success and reaching your goal. When your body goes into fat-burning mode, you teach it to use stored fat as a regular source of energy between meals, and while you sleep. These actions indicate that you are gaining mastery over your metabolism. Some experts say that you should never go hungry on a diet, because it results in killing your metabolism. This is not quite true. Skipping meals is what kills your metabolism, not hunger.

The difference between being hungry and skipping a meal is that one is a signal your body is giving you, while the other is ignoring that signal until a certain period of time has passed. The latter causes your body to shut down and go into starvation mode. Being hungry is a completely natural message that your brain sends out to your body, telling it to eat because your energy stores are low. For this brief period, your body is using and burning fat as a source of energy until you get to your next meal. This may be as little as 15-30 minutes, depending on your activity level for that day. The closer towards the end of that period, the closer your body moves towards skipping a meal and shutting down your metabolism.

Basically, the minute that you feel hungry, is the minute that you should make your way to the fridge! If you are outside of home, then you should have a meal prepared or a planned option to eat somewhere. Preparation is the key here. This preparation is about knowing that you will be hungry soon, and knowing how you will be able to feed your body when the signal hits. You should not be constantly thinking about food, but you should always know how readily accessible your next meal will be. Then, just forget about it until your body gives you the hunger signal.

The more that you listen to your hunger signals, the better you will become at noticing them, and the clearer they will be. Many people have no idea when they are actually hungry or not. This is because they don't listen carefully to their body, so they don't know what their body is telling them. By eating when you are NOT hungry, or not eating when you ARE hungry, you are destroying your body's ability to send you the hunger signal. This signal is just like a muscle. If you don't use it, it becomes weaker. Alternatively, the more you use it, the stronger it becomes. You eventually become so good at reading this signal that you are able to predict how soon it will appear. This skill is a great asset to have when shredding body fat, because it enables you to fuel your metabolism on time, so that it works at its best.

Using and developing the hunger signal is such an important tool, but surprisingly, many authors and experts do not even talk about it. Begin working on using your hunger signal today, by eating as soon as you are hungry and ONLY when you are hungry. Within a couple of days, you will notice how natural this is and how you are working WITH your body, not against it. This will train your body to have an unstoppable metabolism, which in turn, will lead you to obtaining effortless fat-loss.

Cravings

Cravings can be your worst enemy when trying to achieve success on a diet. Many people struggle at fighting their cravings, but there should be no problem if you understand where they come from. Cravings for sweet foods or any other type of food, are almost entirely created as a result of deprivation. Any time you deprive your body of sufficient calories, your body will rebel by sending out signals to over compensate. This usually leads to overindulging in sweet foods or just overeating in general. Not only does the person in this situation become distracted from their weight-loss focus, but he or she usually gains extra weight from the relapse. One step forward, two steps backward.

I want to make sure that you are aware of your cravings and can realize exactly where they come from. With this knowledge, you can quickly dispel any cravings that may occur while you are shredding body fat. There should be no reason to have them at all, because *Shred Body Fat* is not like other diets. *Shred Body Fat* is a lifestyle that feeds your body sufficient food in order to carry out the tasks that fill your day. There is no deprivation involved because your calorie deficit is only be small, while your metabolism continues to remain high. You are merely feeding your body sufficiently, then burning off your meals completely; by using normal daily activity and additional exercise. This will result in small amounts of fat being constantly used as energy in between meals and while you sleep.

Deprivation is the main cause for cravings, but other factors which lead to them can also occur. Being inactive or simply unoccupied during the day can unintentionally put your mind's focus back on food. In order to avoid this, it is important to stay busy. Most people are busy with work, school or family; for the people who are not, a hobby or separate interest may be necessary.

Having more time available can work in your favor if you are focused on your fat-loss goal, but staying busy and occupied throughout the day, can make the weeks go by faster.

Hunger Signals vs Cravings

It is important to know the difference between a food craving and a hunger signal. A hunger signal is there to protect you and make sure that you have food to survive. A food craving is the result of either deprivation or boredom. So how can you decide between the two? Well, with a little practice your hunger signal will be so familiar that you notice it coming before it arrives. Your body will become very good at telling you that it is hungry, and you will get better at hearing it. Soon, it will become a habit to eat when you are hungry, and will feel unnatural to eat when you are not.

You can expect this trigger to work its magic in as little as a day or two. As you continue to follow your hunger signal, it will become stronger and stronger during the days and weeks to come. This process is done naturally by the body, and is something that is rarely talked about by other fitness trainers and health experts. It amazes me that such a fundamental and important idea is completely overlooked by the fitness and diet industry. This basic understanding of your body and being able to listen to its direction, happens to be one of *Shred Body Fat's* little gems. It is so simple yet profound that by ignoring it, you risk setting yourself up for failure. By acknowledging it, success in reaching your desired body weight will seem like the easiest and most natural thing in the world.

In the first day or two of *Shred Body Fat*, your hunger signal may be a little unclear (due to lack of practice). As mentioned previously, this is natural. I cannot stress enough how important it is to be in touch with your body, and listen for the correct signal to eat. This is a skill that you will carry with you for the rest of your life. To further distinguish between a food craving and a hunger signal, I have provided attributes and tips below.

Food Craving

➢ Having a food craving means that you are definitely NOT hungry, but still have a desire to eat food. Food cravings may arrive soon (within 1 hour) after you have already eaten. In this case, you know that you are not hungry, but still preoccupied with food. Get up and go do something. Even if it's just going out to do grocery shopping.

➢ A common cause for a food craving may be that the size of your last meal did not satisfy you. Be aware of this and adjust your meal accordingly next time, so that you are satisfied after you eat.

➢ Drinking a lot water after you have just eaten a meal may leave you feeling bloated. When the bloating goes down, you may feel empty and cravings may occur. For this reason, allow time for your food to digest and avoid drinking water straight after a meal.

➢ Don't eat anything at all until your next meal. It is important to train yourself to eat your meal and then forget about food until you are due to eat again. Avoid nibbling on tiny snacks because this will not only entice you to eat more, but will also affect your next hunger signal.

➢ Beware of chewing gum. The acids in your stomach that occur from a constant flow of saliva in your mouth, can cause a problem. Not only will they entice cravings, but they will also greatly affect your next hunger signal. Apart from this problem, chewing gum can be good for your teeth and clearing your breath. So, I recommend that if you choose to chew gum, do it straight after a meal and stop after about half an hour. This is long before your next hunger signal is due.

Hunger Signal

➢ Depending on the size of your last meal, a hunger signal may vary in the length of time that it takes to occur. After a small meal, your next hunger signal may take 2-3 hours to arrive; after a large meal, the signal may take 4-6 hours to arrive.

➢ A hunger signal can be clearly recognized by the feeling you get inside your stomach. It is completely different to the feeling that you get when you THINK you are hungry. The hunger signal is physical, not mental. It is the difference between thinking you are hungry and knowing you are hungry.

➢ If you are unsure of whether you are hungry or not, try waiting 15 minutes. After 15 minutes, you will know for sure that it's a hunger signal and now time to eat, or that it's just a craving of some sort. Cravings are temporary, which makes them easy to overcome.

➢ With time and practice, you will get good at predicting when your hunger signal will arrive. This with help you to begin preparing for your next meal ahead of time, so that you eat as soon as the signal arrives. It's a beautiful thing.

On the *Shred Body Fat* program, carbohydrate is not converted into fat. Sometimes, you may find yourself in situations where you have no choice but to eat before your hunger signal has arrived. This is not a problem. Just take note and adjust your future meals accordingly. It is most important to stay on-time with your day, schedule and metabolism. This will ensure that you achieve your curfew at the end of the day and get a good night's sleep. As a result, you will be prepared for the next day, and able to continue the process of shredding fat.

Judge Your Portions

As the days pass and you are well into the fat shredding process, you will adjust to the amount of food that you should eat. You will also gain experience and be able to estimate how much food to eat for each particular meal, without counting calories. Naturally, you will be able to judge how much food will keep you energized until your next meal. Remember, you want to be hungry in time for your next meal, so that you will burn fat briefly after the current meal has been burnt off. Then, it is time to recharge your metabolism, by eating immediately. I will discuss exactly how your diet will work, later in this book.

Shred Body Fat consists of 4 meals per day. The second and third meals of the day should not be a problem for decided how much you need to eat. This is because they are larger meals, which will fuel your busiest and most active parts of the day. It is your first and last meals that need a little more attention. Your first meal should give you enough energy to kick-start your day, but must still be compact enough to leave you hungry soon after, around lunchtime. Similarly, your last meal must give you enough energy so that you don't wake up in the middle of the night hungry; while still being compact enough to be burnt off soon after, when you sleep. This will allow your body to go into fat burning mode throughout the night.

Only you will be able to assess your portions of food, because everyone is different. In the next section, I shall make suggestions for meals and basic portion control, but in the end, it is up to you. You need to become familiar with which foods keep you fuller for longer, and adjust the portion sizes to facilitate your meal times. The meal times are only approximate times. You may find that you are hungry earlier or slightly later, but this is fine. Just try to eat soon after you receive the hunger signal. Also, don't be afraid to eat larger portions for lunch and before a gym session. You will need that extra energy to be strong and active during the following hours.

Carbohydrate Portion vs Protein Portion

Measuring macronutrient portions must be treated separately, because carbohydrate and protein both have different roles in the body. In terms of energy, carbohydrate is first and foremost. The body will not even use protein as a source of energy if carbohydrate intake is sufficient. Overdosing on protein will only put a strain on your kidneys and make your body work harder to digest the meal. Therefore, the protein portion in a meal must be considerably smaller than the carbohydrate portion.

A portion of protein consists of between 20-30 grams, where 30 is a maximum and 20 is a minimum. Aiming for a mark of 25g is sensible. This goes for both men and women, despite women needing slightly less protein on a daily basis. Men will favor towards the 30g mark per meal, while women will favor towards the 20g mark. *Shred Body Fat* is not about giving you hard rules and numbers to follow. It is about giving you practical estimates to work with, so that you can use them as a guide. There is nothing difficult about looking at the nutrition label on the packaging of food that you eat, and then measuring a portion that is around the 25 gram mark. That is the way we want it, simple and practical.

Do not concern yourself with misjudging a portion of protein in one particular meal. Your hunger signal will tell you when to eat again, regardless of your protein consumption. The protein in a meal will only contribute to a slower digestion, not the energy intake. This brings us to the carbohydrate portion. The carbohydrate portion has a larger bearing on your energy and the length of time between hunger signals.

A portion of carbohydrate on the *Shred Body Fat* program will consist of 50-100 grams, depending on your gender, size and activity level. This amount is far more flexible than the protein portion. The reason for this is that carbohydrate can be used quite easily by the body. It is always readily available, even when you are just sleeping or watching television. Staying within these amounts may not be as strict, but dropping below 50 grams is not recommended. Shredding body fat is not achieved by cutting calories to a minimum. It is achieved by feeding your body with food, and burning that food off. This allows fat to be utilized. If you continuously feed your body tiny amounts of carbohydrate, you will not be encouraging it to burn anything all. Not even fat. Instead, you will be losing muscle.

Above all things, the most important tool in judging how much to eat, is your hunger signal. This is what you will practice and develop as a way to calculate your portions and your overall food intake. In the beginning, you can use the amounts that I recommend as sensible portions, to guide you; after more time and practice, you won't need to use those amounts anymore. You'll simply acquire an accurate sense and judgment for how much food is enough to get you through to your next meal, before feeling hungry. *Shred Body Fat* becomes tailored specifically to you and your body. In between meals, you must occupy yourself with life and let your body take care of the shredding.

Sleep

Getting enough sleep is vital for shredding body fat. Without proper sleep, your body will shut down and stop burning calories efficiently. Your body and metabolism require approximately 8 hours of sleep per night to function properly. During this 8 hours, your body gets the rest and recuperation it needs to prepare for the following day. While you are following the *Shred Body Fat* program, you should treasure your sleep time. Everything else in this program will be less effective without sufficient sleep. Kick-starting your metabolism with improper sleep, is like trying to start a car with a dead battery.

Besides avoiding a metabolism meltdown, the advantages of getting a good night's sleep are plentiful. The *Shred Body Fat* program requires meal planning, an exercise routine, and listening to your body. Therefore, the energy that you gain from a good night's sleep is essential to staying on the right track. Proper sleep also provides you with the ability to receive the correct hunger signals that your body sends when it needs food. Lack of good sleep will directly interfere with these signals.

47

An effective strategy is to go to sleep at the same time every night and wake up at the same time every morning. Most people do this naturally, but it is definitely the perfect way to set your body clock into a pattern. This will help you to be wide awake throughout the day and then slowly shut down towards bedtime, in a very natural way. Avoid falling asleep with the TV or radio on. Your mind requires complete silence when you sleep, to completely shut down and attain perfect rest. Background noise will only interfere with that. Also, try to make your bedroom as dark as possible. This can add to a great night sleep. A well ventilated room, with clean air is another advantage. By breathing in clean air, you can only induce good sleep. Finally, the temperature of your room should not be too hot or too cold. Having suitable blankets for the state of the room will prevent you from uncomfortably waking up during the middle of the night.

At first, you may only need to make a couple adjustments to your room in order to achieve a great night's sleep. The most important advice I can give you is to have a consistent routine. Be aware of the time when you plan to go to sleep, and prepare for it in advance. This way, you will be ready and your body will be completely relaxed when it is time to close your eyes. Many people stay up late, tiring themselves out by watching TV or doing work. They then go straight to sleep, which does not suit their body too well. Without consciously knowing it, their mind is still partially consumed in the activities prior to sleeping. Avoid doing that. Instead, treat your sleep time as sacred. Your body will respond by providing you with more energy and by keeping your metabolism at full strength.

Once you achieve a metabolism which is always at full strength, your body will develop a habit of shredding fat 24 hours a day. Even when you sleep, you will burn fat. Sleeping is actually very effective for burning fat, because your body is resting, recuperating and has plenty of oxygen to enable fat-loss. When you awake in the morning and eat breakfast, your metabolism is recharged and ready to start the day. The goal here, is to keep shredding fat continuously (24 hours a day), like a machine, until you have your desired body.

Alcohol

Alcohol is not converted into fat by the human body. It is a completely separate entity, in the same way that carbohydrate and fat have no connection. However, there are many drawbacks to consuming alcohol while trying to lose body fat. Alcohol is a toxin. The body uses many resources to burn and remove it. As a result, all other metabolic processes are put on hold. This includes the process of using stored body fat as a source of energy, which is the only way to lose real weight.

The empty calories that alcohol provides, contain no essential vitamins. Furthermore, they require time to be broken down and removed from the body. It's a slow process which delays fat-loss and prevents muscles from receiving quality calories for nourishment. This is why many people feel weak and hung-over on the day after a big night out drinking and partying. Their alcohol consumption puts a tremendous strain on them physically, forcing their energy loss to manifest as a hangover.

Despite alcohol not being converted into fat, people often gain fat easily from it. The reason for this is because the alcohol they drink is usually accompanied by fatty foods. These may include snack foods at a party, or greasy bar food in the form of wings, nachos, fries, etc. Such foods contain high-levels of fat, which is guaranteed to be stored for long periods of time. This is the cause that is attributed to alcohol and weight-gain. By avoiding fatty foods when consuming alcohol, you will maintain the fat-loss that you've previously achieved. It is easy to undo an entire week of fat-loss, with a single night of partying and binging on junk food.

On the flip side, there have been studies done that suggest some alcohol, such as red wine, can reduce the risk of cardiovascular disease. The antioxidants in wine may benefit your health in this way, but the key is moderation. Moderation means a glass of wine with dinner, once or twice a week. Ideally, when you are on the *Shred Body Fat* program; the less alcohol you drink, the better. This will help you to achieve your goal in the shortest amount of time. If you choose to remove alcohol entirely, an improvement in your metabolism will be noticed immediately. The empty calories that were normally consumed will be replaced by stored body fat.

Diet Sodas

Diet sodas contain zero calories due to the artificial sugar that they contain, replacing natural sugar. Regular sodas contain high amounts of sugar, which is why diet sodas are a popular alternative. In most cases, either aspartame or sucralose is the substitute. These artificial sugars have no effect on insulin levels, therefore no calories are digested. Sounds like the perfect solution to quenching your thirst, satisfying your sweet tooth, and avoiding calories all together, right? Not so.

Artificial sweeteners are mostly unnatural substances. Aspartame is an artificial sugar that is in some ways, far more toxic than alcohol. It consists of a molecule which is made up of three components: aspartic acid (40%), phenylalanine (50%), and methyl ester (10%). Aspartic acid is an amino acid which is also an excitotoxin (overstimulates nerve function) that can consistently cross the blood-brain barrier. Phenylalanine is an amino acid, but it is present in abnormally large quantities through the consumption of aspartame. Methyl ester is methyl alcohol (wood alcohol), which is a chemical poison. Methyl ester can also be found in many healthy foods such as fruits and vegetables, but in these foods, it is bound to a substance called pectin. Humans do not carry the enzyme to split pectin from methanol, so in those instances, it passes through the body safely.

Aspartame's sweet taste was discovered in 1965, when a chemist by the name of James Schlatter, happened to spill some on his finger. Soon after, he was shocked to find that it had a pleasant taste, similar to that of sugar. Since that day, artificial sweeteners (such as aspartame) have slowly been introduced to the public and approved by the FDA (*Food and Drug Administration*). Humans are likely to withstand the minor side effects of these artificial sugars, but the long-term neurological dangers may go unnoticed for many years. When the body consumes methyl alcohol alone, as in the case of aspartame, it is broken down and stored as a toxic chemical called formaldehyde. Formaldehyde cannot be removed by the body and is accumulative. That alone, is a serious concern.

The list of symptoms that relate to artificial sweetener intake include severe migraines, skin allergies, memory failure, blackouts, cancer and brain disorders. Astoundingly, brain tumors in America increased by 10% by the end of 1983, which was the first year that *Diet Coke* was released and brought to market. That's some pretty strong circumstantial evidence for the potential danger caused by aspartame. Despite FDA approval, drinks containing aspartame or sucralose have a chemical makeup that cannot be ignored. Such chemicals should not be a part of any health conscious diet.

So, how does this relate to *Shred Body Fat*, you ask? Simply, your liver is an organ that plays a major role in fat metabolism. It is responsible for removing toxins from your body and using fat as energy when needed. Every time you swallow a substance that is toxic, your liver is required to remove it first. This means that instead of digesting fats, it has to deal with removing the unnecessary chemicals that you have presented it with. Therefore, fat metabolism is delayed and restricted. Many people use diet sodas or alcohol as an emotional crutch, but this makes losing fat almost impossible. Even if fat-loss is somehow achieved, muscle-loss will occur.

Your liver is your best friend when shredding body fat. Look after it, keep it clean and avoid exposing it to dangerous chemicals. The result will be that your body will effortlessly burn fat on a daily basis. Also, be aware that diet sodas will contribute to cravings. This is because the body is tricked into consuming something sweet, but without the energy content. Sweetness without energy will lead to desiring the real thing (sugar). Avoid being a slave to food in that way, by simply avoiding diet sodas entirely. Stick to water for quenching your thirst. If you feel like something with a bit more fizz, try Seltzer water (zero calories and zero artificial sugar).

Water

Many people avoid drinking a lot of water because they think it will make them retain fluid and become bloated. In fact, the opposite is true. Insufficient water causes you to become dehydrated. As a consequence, your body is forced to hold on to all the water that it has at that moment. Alternatively, by drinking adequate amounts of water, dehydration is prevented. Your kidneys determine your body's optimal water levels, and flush the excess out of your system. This results in less water retention.

Drinking plenty of water is not only a healthy practice for your body, blood and organs, but it can help to release toxins that build up in your digestive system. These same toxins can make you feel tired and sluggish. Your intestines and colon are very good at storing waste for many days at a time, if you let them. Consuming sufficient amounts water will gradually sweep through and remove this collection of waste from your system. As a result, your bowel movements will become more regular and easier to pass. The effect that water has on your body can be seen and felt within a couple of days. This difference will be obvious by the clarity of your eyes and skin, while feeling more alert and energetic. Other people will also notice the difference in you.

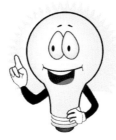

Tip: Drinking too much water with a meal, is not advised. This is because water can dilute gastric juices and interfere with the digestive process. It is fine to sip a little water if your mouth becomes dry while eating, but it is generally best to drink water at least fifteen minutes before a meal. This way, your body will absorb all the nutrients in the food that you eat, by avoiding improper digestion.

Exercise

The most beneficial thing that you can do to kick-start your fat shredding process and raise your metabolism on a daily basis, is exercise. On *Shred Body Fat,* you can reach your desired body weight without exercise, but it will take a lot longer. Exercise can be the difference between reaching your fat-loss goal in a month or two, and reaching it in a year or two. Both are fine, but most people do not want to wait up to two years until they reach their weight-loss goal. Exercise is also responsible for sculpting your body and maintaining muscle, while you are shredding down and losing fat.

Resistance and weight training will keep you burning fat throughout an entire day. The muscle that you build from this training will raise your metabolism for 24 hours a day, 7 days a week. We will get to the resistance and weight training part of *Shred Body Fat,* later in the book. For now, I want to explain the type of exercise that is responsible for directly burning fat. I also want to explain how to apply it, how long to apply it, and what time of day to apply it. These are the key points to remember. Fat burning exercises are simple to apply, but they have to be done in a specific way. Otherwise, you will be wasting your time and achieving very little fat-loss.

Cardio

Cardio is a name that is short for **cardiovascular exercise**. It can be done at different speeds and for different lengths of time. It can also be split up into different variations and combinations, for endurance or heart rate increase. On *Shred Body Fat*, the goal is to use cardio to shred fat directly. We are NOT going to use cardio to increase our metabolism (even though it will do that anyway). So to recap, you will be using cardio to burn fat directly, while using resistance (weight training) to maintain muscle and boost your metabolism.

Cardio = Direct fat-loss

Resistance Training = Indirect fat-loss

Cardiovascular training can include anything that involves movement or an increase in heart rate for a certain period of time. Examples of cardio are: walking, jogging, swimming, dancing, bicycle riding, rowing, cross- country skiing, jumping rope, and aerobics. Almost every sport falls into the category of cardiovascular exercise.

Now, although many of the above activities can provide some benefit to your health and daily energy consumption, very few are great for directly burning fat. The simple explanation for this is that to burn fat, your body requires a good supply of oxygen. Many of the exercises listed above will restrict your oxygen, due to the heart rate increase that is incurred. This leaves you exerting so much energy that your lungs cannot take in a steady, consistent flow of oxygen. Instead, you are left gasping for air while trying to perform such exercises. Basically, any exercise that leaves you short of breath, is not be a good fat-burner.

Choosing an Exercise

A good test for a fat-burning exercise is to see if you can have a normal conversation while doing it. If having a conversation is difficult, this would be because you are breathing heavy during that particular exercise. Therefore, it would not be a good fat-burner. A prime example of an ineffective fat-burner, is swimming. It's a great exercise for keeping fit while raising your metabolism and heart rate, but your breathing is restricted and inconsistent. A swimmer naturally burns a lot of calories during and after the swim, but very little fat is burnt during the actual swim. Jogging is another exercise that is a great exercise for increasing your fitness and metabolism, but again, not good for burning fat directly.

The Perils of Fast Cardio

The biggest mistake that I see people make in the gym or while exercising in general, is doing fast cardio. This is responsible for most people getting very few results, forcing them to eventually give up. So why do people do it? It increases heart rate and raises metabolism for the rest of the day, but unfortunately, it is still an ineffective strategy.

Here's why -

> **Exercising at fast pace does very little for burning fat or building muscle.**

When people tire themselves out by doing fast cardio, it becomes mindless cardio. Firstly, the energy that is spent needs to have more food to fuel it (since stored fat is not being used). This requires more calories to begin with. If insufficient food is provided, the body will begin breaking down muscle tissue as a source of fuel. So, it's a lose/lose situation. Secondly, the metabolism boost that is produced for the rest of the day, usually comes with cravings for larger amounts of food. In most cases, people will justify the increase in calories, with the workout they did. Therefore, the fast-paced cardio usually only provides an outlet for their fast-paced lifestyle.

Compared to resistance training, fast cardio provides little metabolism increase and muscle gain. One resistance training session can increase your metabolism for a few days (due to muscle repair), while a fast cardio boost will only last a few hours. Often, I see injuries relating to joints or strained ligaments from the length of time that people endure at a fast pace. This puts them back even further. If you want to achieve your fat-loss goal in a smart and efficient way, I advise that you stick to resistance training and slow cardio. In the long run, your results will clearly show.

Slow and steady wins the race.

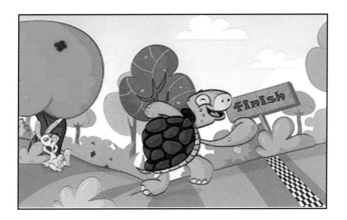

The Best Fat Shredding Exercise

The exercise that I find works best for shredding fat is walking. Walking at a brisk pace that exerts energy, but does not leave you out of breath. This is perfect. The great thing about walking is that it's free. Just select a route in your neighborhood and go! No equipment required, except a good pair of walking shoes. Most people have no problem walking and it doesn't place too much pressure or strain on ligaments or joints. If walking is a problem for you, then riding a bike may be a good alternative. Basically, any exercise will work as long as you keep it at a slow-medium pace. Remember, you must be able to breathe at a steady, consistent rate.

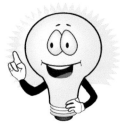

Tip for walkers: Many walkers think that by swinging their arms during a walk, they will be burning more calories. This is not the case. Swinging your arms requires little effort, because they practically move on their own. If anything, swinging your arms will give you momentum and make your walk easier, which is not necessarily a good thing. If you really want to make your walk a challenge, try keeping your hands in your pockets. By doing this, you will find that your legs and hips are doing all the work, which makes the walk a much more productive exercise. If you feel that must make your morning walk even more difficult, try light hand weights or even light leg weights. These will slightly increase the intensity of your cardio. A slight uphill incline also works, but just remember, your cardio should remain low-medium intensity for maximum fat-burning. Your goal is not to build muscle during your cardio workout.

When To Do Cardio

Now that you have chosen your fat-burning exercise, the next step is to do it at the correct time of day. When is the correct time of day? The simple answer is 3-4 hours after you have eaten a meal, depending on its size. During this period, food has been digested and insulin in the blood has cleared. The absolute best time to achieve minimum insulin is when you wake up in the morning. After 8 hours of sleep, your body has been fasting for such a time that almost no insulin is present. This means your body only has a choice of muscle or fat for fuel. If you start your cardio promptly, and keep it at a slow-medium pace (as mentioned above), you will ensure that maximum fat is burnt and minimum muscle is lost. The minimum muscle that you do lose, can be regained through your weight training and a specific meal plan.

If it proves to be impossible for you to fit morning cardio into your daily schedule, an afternoon or night session is fine. Just make sure that it is towards the end of having burnt off your last meal. The reason I advise that morning cardio is the preferred option, is because it's less likely to interfere with your meals and metabolism during the day. Either way, you can avoid any interference by simply planning ahead and being precise. Also, make sure that you eat again straight after you have finished cardio. This is important. The entire *Shred Body Fat* program is very flexible and will accommodate to anyone's schedule, as long as the basics are applied.

Cardio For How Long?

The final part of doing the correct cardio for shredding fat, is committing to a length of time that you will do it for. This is one of the most important parts of *Shred Body Fat*. Let me explain why. It is not until 20 minutes of doing cardio, that your body will start using fat as energy. This is because it takes 20 minutes for fat to leave the fat cell and become fuel for your muscles. Once the fat is being used as fuel, the consistent pace of your fat-burning exercise will burn it at a steady rate. Therefore, 40 minutes of cardio will produce 20 minutes of fat-loss, while 60 minutes of cardio will produce 40 minutes of fat-loss. The longer you do cardio on an empty stomach, the more fat you will burn. Having said that, it is wise to limit your cardio to a maximum of 1 hour 20 minutes. Even this is a little on the lengthy side, compared to 40 minutes or 60 minutes.

You may find that you start with 40 minutes of cardio, twice a week. As you improve your fitness, gradually increase the duration to 60 minutes, and the amount to 3-4 times a week. Whatever you are comfortable with is fine, because you will be moving closer to your fat-loss goal either way. So, how much fat will you be shredding during these cardio sessions?

On the next page, there is a table showing approximately how much fat will be burnt for both women and men.

Fat Burnt During Cardio (grams)

Time	Women	Men
20 mins	0	0
40 mins	7.5	10
60 mins	15	20
80 mins	22.5	30

It's easy to see the grams of direct fat-loss adding up if you dedicate yourself to cardio 3-4 times a week. If you are comfortable with doing even more days of cardio, that is fine too. Just make sure to understand that you are not in a rush to achieve your fat-loss goal. Slow and steady wins the race. Doing too much cardio can make your weight sessions at the gym very difficult, and you may feel that you are losing too much strength or muscle. For this reason, you should be aware that your morning cardio is just one aspect of *Shred Body Fat*. The other parts of the program (meals, weight training, sleep, planning, etc) are just as important. It's a well-rounded machine. If you feel that you risk sacrificing the other components by overdoing it, take a step back and focus on overall consistency. That way, your success is guaranteed.

Start your walk as soon as you wake up

When you wake up after a complete night of sleep, do not waste any time. Try to wake up and be ready to start your morning walk immediately. The best way to do this is by preparing for it the night before. Have everything ready (clothes, shoes, music player, keys, water bottle, etc), so that all you have to do is pick up your stuff and walk out the door. The sooner you start your walk, the sooner you will have finished it. By leaving promptly, you will avoid any hunger pains. This is because your body will become preoccupied with burning fat as your energy source.

You must aim to finish your walk before your stomach realizes that you have not eaten yet. When it finally does realize, you should be home and already preparing your breakfast. How efficient you become at starting your morning cardio, will determine how comfortable you are when during it. If you can be halfway through your walk before you are fully awake, you have done good. If you can make it home and begin eating your breakfast before your hunger signal hits, you have done great. If you happen to completely avoid a hunger signal by the end of your cardio, this is the exception of which you should eat when you are not hungry. After a night of fasting and an hour-long walk on an empty stomach, your body needs food to start your day with energy.

That's a pretty good start to your day. 15-20 grams of fat, gone!

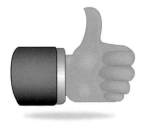

Cardio Recap

To finish up this chapter, I'm going sum up the main points that create a perfect fat-burning cardiovascular exercise. These will make it easier for you to decide if the exercise that you are doing is actually burning fat.

✓   It is low-intensity (slow-medium pace)

✓   It is done on an empty stomach

✓   It is lasting longer than 20 minutes

✓   It is continuous throughout (no stopping)

Starvation Mode

When your body is not fed food periodically, it goes into shut-down. This shut-down is called starvation mode. Whenever you become hungry, your body is telling you to eat because it requires energy. The very last of your carbohydrate stores are reserved for the brain, while your body and its muscles use stored fat for fuel. Muscle tissue also becomes vulnerable to being broken down as a source of energy.

As hunger worsens, the body begins to increase the ratio of muscle for fuel against fat. This continues until finally your body enters starvation mode and stops burning fat altogether. *Shred Body Fat* avoids starvation mode like *The Plague*. The main focus of this book is on burning a little fat, as often as possible, while rebuilding the muscle that is sacrificed. This muscle is rebuilt through resistance training and correct nutrition.

Shred Body Fat Focus

- Burn a little fat often

- Rebuild muscle lost

Many uninformed nutritionists preach that once your body reaches starvation mode, your body will turn food into fat. This is simply not the case. De Novo Lipogenesis is still an unlikely scenario once starvation mode is reached, but your metabolism will become much slower to utilize food as energy thereafter. Your metabolism will need to be rebuilt.

Calories In vs Calories Out

On *Shred Body Fat*, carbohydrate will not be converted to body fat. Instead, it will be the energy source that is used to fuel your metabolism. Eating a fat-free diet means that even a surplus in carbohydrate intake will still result in less overall fat storage. This is because you won't be directly storing fat from high-fat foods, to begin with. It is a basic concept that is the platform for your entire meal plan. Excess carbohydrate will be used to increase strength and muscle, until it is finally burn off through body heat.

Having this understanding is beneficial towards your choices in food. Your first goal in *Shred Body Fat* is to avoid storing fat. This is accomplished through your diet. Your second goal is to shred the fat that you already have stored around your body. This is accomplished in two ways - 1) cardio on an empty stomach 2) energy used between meals. The latter is a result of your metabolism using your fat stores as fuel. Despite enabling your metabolism to continue working, fat is used only for a brief period, before you shift into starvation mode.

For simply maintaining your body weight, a small surplus in carbohydrate can work well, provided your fat intake is kept to a minimum. *Shred Body Fat* is not about maintaining body weight. *Shred Body Fat* is about losing body weight (in the form of fat). Therefore, a calorie surplus will not work. There must be a calorie deficit. This grants your body permission to briefly use stored body fat, after it has burnt off your last meal. Body fat is only used as energy until you feed yourself again, or go into starvation mode.

The message that I want you to understand is this: To shred body fat throughout the day, you must have more calories going out than coming in. The calories coming in are the ones that your body uses as primary energy, in the form of carbohydrate. You will achieve a calorie deficit simply by controlling your portions, burning off your meals, and listening to your hunger signals. There is no need to count (or cut) calories.

Every time you get the <u>Hunger Signal</u>, you know two things:

1. You are burning fat as energy.

2. You don't have much time before you

go into starvation mode. Time to eat!

For Women

I feel that it is important to write a section in this book just for women, on the subject of shredding body fat. This is because women and men usually have different goals. Men tend to be more focused on building muscle, size and strength; while women generally stay focused on having a slim, toned, less muscular physique. A gym scenario can be an intimidating experience for a woman, especially if the room is filled will a bunch of "dudes" lifting heavy weight. For this reason, many women prefer to join a gym which allows only female members. Other women simply feel more comfortable physically when working out in a single-sex gym.

Shred Body Fat is a book written for both men and women. The principles of shredding body fat do not discriminate between genders. They are the same for 99.9% of humans. Men may have slightly faster metabolisms (due to carrying more weight, size and muscle mass), but this only accounts for a slightly faster fat-loss rate. Remember, even though men have faster metabolic rates, they must eat more food in order to support their metabolism. More food means a higher fat intake, even if they are restricting fat in their diets (most carbohydrates and proteins contain a small amount of fat). So, a man's higher metabolic rate only gives him a slight advantage in losing body fat.

Although the cover of this book may be intimidating to some people (especially women), the focus still remains on teaching all people how to remove stored fat from their bodies. This includes both genders equally. The principles are based on science and the way that the human body uses fat as an energy source. The diet and exercise program in this book applies to women just as much as it applies to men. When doing resistance training, women should simply lift a weight that challenges their own personal strength. The only person you are in competition with is yourself.

As a woman, you will find that you become more aware of your strength capabilities. Your body fat percentage will go down, as a reward for your efforts. Throughout this book, I have made references to weight training and putting on unwanted muscle-mass. I will make this very clear, and reiterate that weight training alone will NOT make you bigger. Weight training will only serve to break down muscle tissue and repair it so that it becomes stronger. Much like breaking a bone. It repairs and becomes stronger with time. The muscle strength that you build will serve to keep your metabolism and fat shredding process at its peak.

If you are unfamiliar with resistance training, start slow and take time to become familiar with your body. Don't be afraid to watch others and ask for help on how to use a machine or exercise. After a few sessions, your body will adjust and become stronger. Resistance and weight training is just one tool that you will use to shred fat. There are many other tools in this book that require your focus and persistence, in order to reach your fat-loss goal. In many ways, this book is suited to women, because it encourages you to spend minimum time in the gym. Basically, you should find an exercise that best works the muscle which you intend to strengthen, then do it with a weight that challenges you. Your sessions should be short but challenging, therefore requiring very little time to complete.

Fiber

For people who do not know about fiber, this section will explain what it is and the advantages of implementing it into your diet. Fiber is found in many foods, especially those of plant origin. It is the part of food which cannot be digested, so it passes directly through you. The body lacks the necessary enzymes to break fiber down. For this reason, it can be consumed and released from the body relatively fast. In the process, it may also remove digested food, water, and toxins. The benefits of a diet high in fiber are directly related to intestinal health and bowel regularity. These can even help prevent colon cancer, by reducing the amount of time that food and potential cancer-causing agents sit inside the colon.

People who suffer from high blood-cholesterol can also benefit from a high-fiber diet. Bad cholesterol (LDL) can be eliminated by bile acids in the intestines, which cling to fiber, and are then removed from the body. This reduces LDL levels in the blood. Diabetics can delay blood-sugar by eating high-fiber. Their result is a reduction in blood-sugar spikes, and a slower sugar release into the bloodstream. This fiber balance, combined with eating low GI (Glycemic Index) foods, can have a tremendous effect in the life of someone who is looking to improve their energy levels.

The benefits of a high-fiber diet can also play an important role in fat-loss. Foods containing fiber are generally larger, more filling foods, with a high water content. This means that their calories are fewer, compared to other foods of the same volume. Also, their chewing time is longer, while their bulk fills the stomach much sooner. Basically, the time that you spend eating is increased, but without the additional calories. This leads to greater enjoyment and satisfaction from your meals.

There are 2 types of fiber: Soluble and Insoluble. These two categories are based on their solubility of water. *Insoluble fibers* create a soft bulk, which assists the removal of waste products within the intestinal passage. They also help prevent hemorrhoids, constipation and colon cancer. *Soluble fibers* form a gel, which slows down stomach emptying and can keep you fuller for longer. These fibers can also reduce bad cholesterol, by binding and excreting bile acids; while regulating blood sugar, by way of sugar absorption within the intestines. This is perfect for diabetics or people who are trying to lose weight, provided calories are not too low.

Foods that are high in fiber also contain vitamins and minerals that the body needs. All types of fiber can contribute to a healthy diet, whether they are soluble or insoluble. My advice is to have a good variety and continuously feed your body sufficient amounts. **Warning:** There is such a thing as eating too much fiber. Too much fiber may leave you with excess bloating, gas, and having to run to the bathroom constantly. As a result, your body may not absorb valuable nutrients from the food you eat. Approximately 30 grams of fiber per day is adequate, but this can vary from person to person. Listening to your body, observing your regularity (bowel movements) and gauging how you feel, can help you to adjust your fiber intake accordingly.

Below is a list of foods to include in your diet which contain fiber.

Fruits & Vegetables	Serving Size	Soluble Fiber (g)	Insoluble Fiber (g)	Total Fiber (g)
Apple (skin included)	1 medium	2.2	1.0	3.2
Banana	1 medium	2.1	0.7	2.8
Orange	1 medium	2.1	1.3	3
Pear	1 medium	0.8	3.2	4
Plums	1 medium	0.6	0.5	1.1
Artichoke (cooked)	1 medium	4.7	1.8	6.5

Asparagus (cooked)	1/2 cup	1.7	1.1	2.8
Broccoli, raw	1/2 cup	1.3	1.4	2.7
Brussels sprouts	1 cup	1.7	1.9	3.6
Carrot, raw	1 medium	1.1	1.5	2.6
Green peas (cooked)	1/2 cup	3.2	1.2	4.4
Potato (skin included)	1 medium	2.4	2.4	4.8
Sweet potato (peeled)	1 medium	2.7	2.2	4.9
Tomato	1 medium	0.3	1	1.3
Zucchini (cooked)	1/2 cup	1.4	1.2	2.6

Whole Grains	Serving	Soluble	Insoluble	Total
Barley (cooked)	1/2 cup	3.3	0.9	4.2
Brown rice (cooked)	1/2 cup	1.3	0.1	1.4
Oatmeal (cooked)	1 cup	2.4	1.6	4.0
Popcorn (air popped)	1 cup	1	0.2	1.2
Pumpernickel bread	1 slice	1.5	1.2	1.7

Rye bread	1 slice	1.9	0.8	2.7
Wheat bran	1/2 cup	11.3	1.0	12.3
Wheat germ	2 tbsp.	2.2	0.4	2.6
Whole grain bread	1 slice	2.8	0.1	2.9
Whole wheat bread	1 slice	1.6	0.3	1.9
Whole grain pasta	2 cups	8.2	4.4	12.6

Nuts, Seeds & Beans	Serving	Soluble	Insoluble	Total
Almonds, raw	1 ounce	0.7	3.5	4.2
Black beans (cooked)	1/2 cup	3.8	3.1	6.9
Kidney beans (cooked)	1/2 cup	2.9	2.9	5.8
Lentils (cooked)	1/2 cup	2.8	3.8	6.6
Pinto beans (cooked)	1/2 cup	5.5	1.9	7.4
Psyllium husks	2 tbsp.	7.1	0.9	8.0
Split peas (cooked)	1/2 cup	1.1	2.4	3.4

As you can see, many of the foods listed are fruits, vegetables and whole grains or whole wheat. These are easy to select when doing your grocery shopping. Changing to these foods is a step in the right direction for your health and well-being, more so than your fat-loss. Having said that, you health is closely related to your body weight and body fat. Maintaining a health conscious attitude will keep you attentive to your body's best interests, which is the foundation of *Shred Body Fat*. As you sculpt the outside of your body, why not enhance the inside at the same time? Your overall health on this program is the real result that you will be receiving at the end. It's all about having the respect and understanding of how your body works and how it should be treated. Having the shredded body that you may desire, will simply be the icing on the cake.

3. Diet (battle plan)

Traditional Diets

Traditional diets and nutritional advice will have you believe that if you burn more calories than you consume, your body will lose fat due to a calorie deficit. They will also have you believe that the reverse is true; if you consume more calories than you burn each day, you will store the surplus and gain fat. These are both very simplistic yet ineffective ways of looking at fat-loss and fat-gain. The important missing factor is how different macronutrients work in different ways within a normal, healthy diet. Therefore, it is not as simple as calculating the calories taken in and the calories sent out as energy.

Firstly, eating less calories in an unorganized way, will promote a slow metabolism and muscle-loss. By cutting carbohydrate intake too much, you will send your body into starvation mode. The body is then forced to use the protein and fat in a meal as energy, which is a delayed process. While this is happening, muscle is broken down to be converted into carbohydrate and used as fuel. The whole process spells disaster for long-term fat loss. Secondly, eating more calories in the form of carbohydrate will promote fat storage from the fat within a meal, but if zero fat is in the meal to begin with, those extra calories will be used for muscle growth or will be eventually burnt off through body heat.

In both of the cases above, no support is given to the calories-in versus calories-out bodyweight theory. What needs to be understood is that when a diet is manipulated in an irregular way to promote fat-loss, the body is put under tremendous strain to compensate for this change. Muscle-loss almost always occurs during an unnatural process. Equally important to know, is that when a human is fed surplus calories of a good nature, he or she can avoid fat storage simply by using the body's inability to create De Novo Lipogenesis.

Now, *Shred Body Fat* does not recommend that you go and eat crazy amounts of carbohydrate just because it will not turn to fat. Instead, it recommends that you use this knowledge in a smart and practical way to achieve a balanced diet. This will force your body to use carbohydrate as energy and burn stored fat in between meals. On the next page, is a table that shows how the body uses food after a meal.

Meals contain: *Carbohydrate, Protein, Fat and Alcohol.*

Carbohydrate	⇒	Stored as glycogen and used immediately after eating.
Protein	⇒	Broken down into amino acids and sent for muscle repair.
Fat	⇒	Stored and used as energy after carbohydrate is depleted.
Alcohol	⇒	Puts all other processes on hold, until toxin is burnt off.

As you can see from the table above, the process is quite simple and normal until alcohol enters the equation. Alcohol is a toxin that needs to be removed from the body and burnt off before the others. While this is happening, everything is put on hold, including the body's metabolism.

Your Objective

If I could sum up the entire *Shred Body Fat* program in one sentence it would be this: A balanced meal plan that revolves around completely burning off your meals, smart exercise and proper sleep. There is one factor that the balanced meal needs to account for when shredding fat from your waistline or anywhere else around your body. It needs to have a deficit in your intake of daily fat. Many will argue that the body needs fat and it is unhealthy to do this, but I am not talking about removing healthy fats from your diet. I am talking about unhealthy fats and excess fats, which are responsible for stopping your fat-loss progress.

In achieving a diet which eliminates all bad fats as well as excess fats from your meals, we face a challenge. Most people are not knowledgeable to the point where they know what types of fat in food are entering their body. So, the easiest and best strategy that I find works for everyone is this:

> **Eat a fat-free diet, then add good fats through supplements or certain foods.**

This simplifies your diet by removing ALL fats, but still allows you to manually add the essential fats that your body needs, to function in a healthy manner. By wiping out all fat and starting from scratch, you allow yourself to burn stored body fat as a source of energy; while still receiving good fats separately through supplements, e.g. fish oil, safflower oil and flaxseed oil. Doing this until you feel confident in your food selection skills will make your diet easy to figure out.

The reason I find this strategy to work best is because a tailored fat-free diet is very easy for anyone to create. It only involves removing fat from your meals, and this can be as simple as looking at nutrition labels and the fat content in foods that you buy. Paying attention to the way a meal is cooked or prepared may also be necessary. Grilling or broiling is always a better option than frying or deep-frying your food. Purchasing a book which contains the fat-count for different foods, can also help you to identify high amounts of fat.

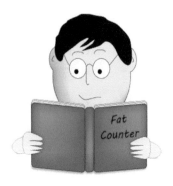

Removing fat from your diet is only a slight adjustment and shouldn't affect your taste in food too much. Most of my clients do not even notice the change. The missing fat can easily be replaced by adding flavor from various non-fat sauces, herbs, spices, or vinegars. Eating a fat-free diet is the foundation of the *Shred Body Fat* program. You will simply be replacing the fat that you used to use as a secondary source of energy from food, with the fat from your belly or your hips. You can get creative with it and prepare fat-free meals that still taste great. This will turn out to be a small price to pay for the lean, shredded body that awaits you.

Fat-free Diet

What I described above is effectively known as a "Fat-free Diet," but it does not really eliminate all fats; just the bad ones! Obviously, you cannot take every gram of fat out of your diet (because most carbohydrates and protein contain at least 1 or 2 grams of fat), but try to keep each meal around or under the 5 gram mark. The reason this constitutes a "Fat-free diet" is because you are taking 99% of the added fat from your diet, while adding back the essentials. The next step is to buy Omega-3 and Omega-6 from your local health store and implement it as part of your diet.

Eating a Fat-free diet is simple once you get used to what you need to look for. It is much easier than cutting carbs from your diet and is much healthier too. The only thing it requires from you, is a basic understanding of foods and how they are prepared. You don't have to be overly picky, but you do have to be selective. With time, you will become good at choosing your foods and choosing how to cook them. You will also be able to avoid fatty dressings and condiments, such as mayonnaise. Get into the habit of looking at labels and recognizing the amount of fat in all foods that you purchase from the store.

What Does A Meal Contain?

It can be difficult to know what a balanced meal should look like. *Shred Body Fat* removes fat entirely from your diet (meal plan), then adds essential fats back, in the form of supplements. Despite eliminating all other fat manually, almost every food has some trace of fat. This accounts for the 1-5 grams of fat that most meals contain naturally, and cannot be avoided. These meals are still a part of a fat-free diet, because their fat is so minimal. Meals that have 5-10 grams, fall into the low-fat category.

Meals Containing Fat

0-5 grams	Fat-free
5-10 grams	Low-fat
10-15 grams	Regular meal
15+ grams	High-fat

Now, the rest of the meal will contain a healthy balance between carbohydrate and protein. This does not mean that they will be equal amounts or even equal portion sizes. Remember, on a normal diet, protein will not be used as energy. Its purpose is to provide the body with nutrients and amino acids, not to be burnt as fuel. Excess protein serves no purpose. It will only put stress on the kidneys, before being removed from the body. Therefore, a balanced meal shall consist of a portion of protein that is much smaller than the portion of carbohydrate.

On *Shred Body Fat*, if we take a meal containing 100 grams worth of macronutrients, the split should be as follows: 70 grams of carbohydrate, 25 grams of protein, and 5 grams of fat. This would supply approximately 3-4 hours worth of energy, depending on your activity levels during that period. These are just estimations which are made to give you an idea about how a meal should appear. It is clear that carbohydrate is the heart of the meal, allowing your body to use it as primary fuel; while protein and fat are secondary, so as to serve their purpose.

On the next page, there is a pie chart which displays the ratio of a meal, as a percentage. This example works well for a meal consisting of macronutrients which total 100 grams. Again, these are just approximate figures that will give you an idea of what your meal should contain. When the overall size of the meal is larger, it is usually the carbohydrate portion that should be increased, not the protein or fat. Carbohydrate requirements are determined by your future activity levels. In other words, if you know that you are going to the gym after you eat, you should increase the carbohydrate in your meal accordingly. The pie graph may not resemble what your plate of food should look like (because different foods have different calorie density), but as a general guide, it works.

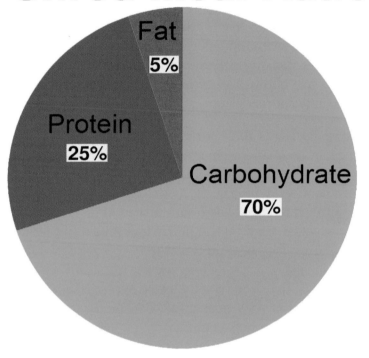

Note: *The fat percentage does not include essential fats that you add to your meal separately. It only accounts for the minimal fat that cannot be avoided. This fat is found naturally in most lean protein and carbohydrate.*

Don't Bother Counting Calories

The reason that calorie counting simply does not work, is because everyone is different, and everyone requires a different calorie intake. With so many changes in metabolism during the day and so many fluctuations in activity levels, you would have to be a mathematical genius to calculate how many calories are required. This is even without including the fact that each type of macronutrient is responsible for different tasks in the body, while consuming and distributing energy in different ways. It's safe to say that with so many factors to consider, your exact calorie requirements are impossible to predict. Counting and measuring calories will only distract you from your real focus.

On *Shred Body Fat* the calorie-counters that you will use are your hunger signals and your attention to portion control. Your portions should be adjusted to the time of day and your activity levels. As mentioned previously, your experience will help you decide how much food will keep you satisfied until your next meal. It is okay to look at the time and notice how long it has been since you last ate. This can help you to prepare for your next meal and give you an idea of when your next hunger signal will be arriving. Just make sure that you don't obsess over the clock or find yourself waiting for your next meal. Constantly thinking about your next meal will not help your natural hunger signal occur. Just look at the clock once if you have to, then occupy yourself with other tasks.

It is also important that you develop a basic understanding of what a meal consists of. In a nutshell, a meal should consist of carbohydrate for energy, and protein for meal balance. Protein is not used as a source of energy. It simply controls your blood sugar levels during digestion, before being transported to other areas of the body for muscle recovery. Protein will help you feel fuller for longer, but it is the carbohydrate in a meal that we shall focus on. Carbohydrates are the real calories that will feed your body the energy it needs. This energy will be used for general muscle use and daily activity.

Control Portions

Controlling your portions simply means preparing sufficient food to last you until your next meal, but no longer. The better that you become at doing this, the better you will be at shredding fat throughout the day; just be careful not to leave yourself short of energy. Make sure you eat enough to feel great and to be active during your day. Eating too fewer calories will drag your metabolism down and send you into starvation mode. When this happens, your fat shredding will slow down to a snail's pace.

Sabotaging your metabolism is the worst thing that you can do to yourself and it must be avoided. Make sure you do not wait too long to eat, but also make sure that you eat only when you are hungry. This is very important. Eating only when you are hungry is as much responsible for a fast metabolism as eating sufficient food. They both work together. When you develop a pattern of eating, burning, and then eating again; your body turns into a fat-burning furnace. Your eating plan must be managed in this way. Staying active during the day helps the process, but having the correct portions that you personally require, is crucial.

What you must practice is judging your portions so that they are large enough to supply plenty of energy to your body and metabolism; however, still controlled in size so that you will be hungry in 3 to 4 hours. **There is no need to count calories here**. As you become accustomed to the food that you prepare for yourself, you will be able to judge how much is necessary. You will also gain experience from knowing how easily you burnt off the previous meals that you prepared, and at what time of day they were burnt off. Considering the time of day is always important. This is because you will naturally burn more calories during the middle of the day, as opposed to the evening, when you are less active.

Lean Protein

When selecting the protein that is going to complete your meal, it is important to not only pick good sources, but to also pick lean sources. It goes without saying that a fat-free diet includes lean protein. Many sources of protein that are found in meals, are accompanied by high levels of fat or saturated fat. Therefore, you must choose your protein wisely and also choose how it is cooked or prepared. Below is a list of great protein sources, which can be included in your diet. All meats should be trimmed of fat, prior to cooking.

* Chicken breast

* Venison

* Turkey breast

* Egg whites

* Fish

* Shellfish

* Non-fat milk

* Whey powder

* Lean beef

From the list above, two of the proteins should have strict portion control. These are: beef (due its saturated fat content) and salmon (due its overall fat content). Beef is a great source of iron, so it should still remain in your diet. It can be eaten 1-2 times a week. Salmon is a great source of essential fatty acids, so it should also remain (2-3 times per week).

Adding Good Fats

As mentioned before, the easiest and most simple way to add good fats to your diet is through supplements. Many foods contain good fats, but also contain bad fats. Salmon is a prime example. It is a great source of Omega-3 fatty acids, but it also contains saturated fat which will be stored as body fat. Some of my clients tell me that they eat salmon all the time, because they were under the impression that it only contains good fats. Unfortunately, they then struggle to figure out why they are not losing weight. I tell them that salmon is great, but must be eaten in moderation. It certainly should not be your prime source of Omega-3 supplementation.

Two of the best supplements that you can add to your diet are fish oil and flaxseed oil. Fish oil normally comes in capsules, which are easy to take with meals. Flaxseed oil usually comes in liquid form, and can be sprinkled over your breakfast cereal or taken straight. A word of warning though, these healthy fats should not be used in cooking or placed under high heat temperatures. This is because extreme heat will destroy good fats, and turn them into bad fats. Canola oil and olive oil are the best oils for cooking. Just be sure to use them as a spray, to minimize the oil content in your cooking.

Foods such as avocados and nuts contain monounsaturated fats which can lower bad cholesterol (LDL) in the bloodstream, while protecting the good cholesterol (HDL). This can only occur if these monounsaturated fats replace the saturated fats in your diet. Remember, too much of any good fat will be stored as body fat and will need to be burnt off. So, control your intake of good fats for optimal health and optimal fat-loss.

Calcium

Calcium is a mineral that is essential to bones, teeth, nerve function, muscle function, cardiovascular health, circulatory health, and blood clot prevention. It also acts as an enzyme regulator. Many fitness experts will drill a hole into your brain by talking about the importance of protein for muscle growth, after a workout. Unfortunately, they won't mention a word about calcium and its relevance to your fitness and strength. Any time you lift a weight or are involved in strenuous activity, your bones are subjected to the force and intensity of the exercise. In the same way that your muscles need to be repaired after heavy lifting, so do your bones.

Bone strength will occur in the same way as muscle strength occurs from being fed carbohydrate and protein. Although, to feed your bones, you will be using quality calcium. The calcium in your diet alone, will not be sufficient for maximum bone growth and strength. This is because many foods (such as milk) have plenty of calcium, but are unable to be absorbed well by the body. I recommend taking *Calcium Citrate* or *Coral Calcium*, with vitamin D and Magnesium for best absorption. *Calcium Carbonate* is a cheaper form of calcium with less absorption. Avoid it.

The best time to take calcium is with your food, straight after a workout. This allows your bones to be fed immediately after physical exertion, in the same way that your muscles would be fed post-workout. Take between 500-1000mg. The long-term result of taking a calcium supplement directly after a workout, is that your bones will become denser and stronger. This will enable you to lift more weight, and add to your metabolism. Increasing your bone strength is what will give you an enormous advantage in the gym, while you continue to shred fat.

Multivitamin

Without going into too much unnecessary detail about supplements, I will mention one more thing. Do yourself a favor and take a multivitamin every morning with breakfast. After eight hours of sleeping and possibly one hour of cardio, there is a good chance that your body will not get all the vitamins and minerals that it is lacking, during your breakfast. To compensate for this, a multivitamin will do the job. For something that takes so little time, it can prove to be a valuable investment in your health.

The short-term benefits can include increased energy, stress reduction, and enhanced immune function. The long-term benefits include cardiovascular health, decreased risk of osteoporosis, improved eye health and brain function. I find that people who do not take a multivitamin everyday, are usually the same people who often become run-down or sick with the flu. Neither of these symptoms are fun. So, avoid these outcomes and keep your health intact, by taking a multivitamin religiously. Even the cheapest multivitamin on the store shelf, usually contains most of your daily needs.

On *Shred Body Fat*, a clear and noticeable difference will be felt by you when taking a multivitamin and calcium supplement. If you feel the need to take extra vitamins or supplements that you are used to taking, this is fine. Just make sure they do not become something that you depend on. Naturally, women may also consider an Iron supplement. *Shred Body Fat* is about living a normal, healthy lifestyle without the need for too many extras. I put the above two supplements (multivitamin and calcium) into the essentials category, alongside the essential fatty acids (Omega-3 and Omega-6) that your brain and body relies on, to function perfectly.

The Meal Plan

The meal plan for *Shred Body Fat* is what I believe to be one of the simplest plans to have ever been created. The name "meal plan" is just another term to replace "diet," but in this case, diet is not a fair description. Your *Shred Meal Plan* will not have the fundamental errors that most diets have. Plus, it will not make false promises. Just about every other weight-loss program in the last 30 years has made false promises. This meal plan will use basic science to shred fat. How this is achieved is by feeding the body all the energy and nutrients it needs, while still creating a minor surplus in calories. Your focus will be on feeding your body well enough, so that in between meals, fat stores are used as energy. No food cravings will occur, because you will be feeding your body with satisfying portions. You will then be generating your own REAL hunger signals, which will only happen when your body requires a meal. Planning and timing is critical; you must aim to make them a habit. This will program your body perfectly, so that it uses food as energy and burns stored fat as a reserve.

6 Meals (not a good idea)

For some years now, many weight-loss gurus advocate a meal plan based around the idea of having 6 smaller meals per day, rather than the traditional 3 larger meals. The theory is that the smaller meals become more frequent, and when consumed in between your daily chores, your metabolism speeds up as a result. What the weight-loss gurus do not explain, are the complications that come from eating 6 smaller meals every day. These are responsible for long-term weight-loss failure.

Firstly, who has time to prepare 6 meals per day and stop to eat them in between work, school or play? I'm not saying it can't be done (I have even tried it myself), but it is extremely inconvenient and impractical. Secondly, a much greater problem arises, which should be your primary concern. Eating 6 small meals a day will never leave you feeling satisfied. You will always feel like you are eating less than your body needs, because your meals are so small, despite being more frequent. The main purpose of a successful diet should be to keep you burning fat, without deprivation. If you feel that you are deprived of food, your diet fails and you will eventually fail too. So, the number 1 focus should be on eating enough food so that it doesn't effect your mood or your day in a negative way. This is the true indication that your diet or meal plan can be successful.

Shred Meal Plan

Introducing the *Shred Body Fat* meal plan. The beauty of this meal plan is that you eat 4 times per day, which still lifts your metabolism, but without disrupting your day. This allows you to focus on other things. You want to be busy and occupied during your day, so that you are not constantly thinking about food. Instead, you want to be burning it! As discussed previously, there is a misconception that the more meals you eat, the faster your metabolism will be. Not so. What is far more responsible for speeding up your metabolism is: actually burning off your meals and then eating promptly, when your hunger signal arrives. Timing is the key.

It is important to make sure that your day commands your meal plan, not the other way around. You should be busy and active during the day, while eating ONLY when you are hungry or due for a meal. Sometimes you may be so busy that you forget you are hungry. When this happens, your brain may distract you from your hunger signal. With practice, you will overcome this by knowing instinctively that it is time to eat. You will know that you have definitely burnt off your last meal and your body is ready for refueling, despite being occupied with other things. In most cases though, your hunger signal will rarely fail you.

Below, you can see a simple diagram that displays how your day should progress and how your *Shred Meal Plan* will fit into your day.

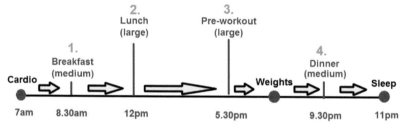

The *Shred Meal Plan* is structured in a way that you use the busiest parts of your day to burnt off your larger meals. This helps you to burn more fat in between your meals. Then, after a long day, your body sleeps for a minimum of 8 hours for full recovery. Your body will continue to burn fat, because you are in full fat-burning mode while you sleep.

In the diagram above, the size of your meals are indicated by the vertical blue lines. Your two largest meals are in the middle of the day, while your two medium meals are for breakfast and dinner. The reason that I describe them as medium is because they are only slightly smaller than the larger meals. The medium meals will provide you with energy for about 3 hours, while the larger meals will provide for about 4-5 hours. These are just basic guidelines, which are not exact. They are there to show you how to easily fit 4 complete meals into your day, with activity in between those meals. Notice that your first large meal (lunch) will be burnt by mild activity, during a 5-hour period; while your second large meal will be burnt by heavier activity in the gym, during a 4-hour period.

Many people make the mistake of eating a breakfast that is too small (coffee with a piece of toast). Or even a dinner that too small, because they feel they should not eat before bedtime. In both cases, you need more food than less. Your breakfast is what kick-starts your metabolism and day, while your dinner is what prepares you for the next 8-10 hours without food, during your night of sleep. Your dinner is also responsible for the repair work that your body needs at the end of your day. For these reasons, the *Shred Meal Plan* has both breakfast and dinner as medium-sized meals.

Breakfast needs to be a sufficient size to boost your day, but still compact enough so that you are hungry for your second meal around midday. Dinner also needs to be a sufficient size to feed your body after the gym workout. It must aid your recovery throughout the night, but still be compact enough to avoid leaving you bloated before sleeping. You want to encourage your body to shred fat throughout the night by having burnt off your dinner after a few hours into your sleep. This way, fat will become your source of energy for the remainder of the night, as you sleep. If you decide to do cardio when you wake up, your dinner may affect how you feel when you rise. Take this into account.

Experiment with what works best in the first week, and adjust accordingly. If you can master this part of your day, your success will be assured. It really depends on the timing and planning of your meals, as well as the preparation for your sleep curfew and early morning cardio. Your sleep curfew is something that will ensure you get your full 8 hours of sleep. This will be responsible for how you feel the next day.

Beware of Low-fat

The terms "low-fat" and "light" can be very misleading. Do not make the mistake of assuming that they are the correct choices. Companies can use these words to promote products as a healthy alternative, when really they are just a healthier alternative to their regular product. Many "low-fat" or "light" products can still contain levels of fat that will restrict your ability to lose weight. In some cases, you may even find that you gain weight, because the low-fat content is relative to the serving size, which happens to be very small. By misjudging servings, meals can equate to high amounts of fat.

Another problem to be aware of in "low-fat" or "light" products is the type of fat involved. Some products may claim to be lower in fat, but end up having saturated or trans fats as their entire fat content. These should be avoided, even if they come in small doses. The fat-free (non-fat) option is always better, and will eliminate any disguises that low-fat foods present.

Nutrition Labels and Serving Sizes

It is important to understand what to look for when reading nutrition facts and ingredients. I have mentioned previously in this book that trans fats can be hidden under various names, and they must be avoided. The only way to find these is by looking at the list of ingredients in the food product that you are buying. Apart from trans fats, other nutritional information is quite easy to read, as long as you know what to look for on the nutrition label. A product that might appear to be low-fat, may actually be a bad choice. Take a look at the nutrition label for whole milk, on the next page.

Nutrition Facts

Serving Size 244 g

Amount Per Serving

Calories 146	Calories from Fat 71

	%Daily Value
Total Fat 8g	12%
Saturated Fat 5g	23%
Trans Fat	
Cholesterol 24mg	8%
Sodium 98mg	4%
Total Carbohydrate 13g	4%
Dietary Fiber 0g	0%
Sugars 13g	
Protein 8g	

Vitamin A	5%	•	Vitamin C	0%
Calcium	28%	•	Iron	0%

*Percent Daily Values are based on a 2,000 calorie diet. Your daily values may be higher or lower depending on your calorie needs.

Figure 1

Whole milk is considered to be a fairly nutritious food (provided you are not lactose intolerant). In Figure 1, you can see there is a healthy supply of protein, carbohydrate, and even calcium. The calorie supply is kept to a modest amount of 146. There is a little sodium and cholesterol also, but this is not the problem that you should be concerned about. Look at the fat content. There are 8 grams of total fat, which contain 5 grams of saturated. Now, look at the serving size. 244 grams is equal to one cup of milk. It is clear that for one small serving of milk, 8 grams of fat (5 saturated) is too much. Your body will store this 8 grams and will have to burn it off before it starts to shred the fat that you already have.

Nutrition Facts

Serving Size 245 g

Amount Per Serving	
Calories 83	Calories from Fat 2

	%Daily Value
Total Fat 0g	0%
Saturated Fat 0g	1%
Trans Fat	
Cholesterol 5mg	2%
Sodium 103mg	4%
Total Carbohydrate 12g	4%
Dietary Fiber 0g	0%
Sugars 12g	
Protein 8g	

Vitamin A	10%	Vitamin C	0%
Calcium	31%	Iron	0%

*Percent Daily Values are based on a 2,000 calorie diet. Your daily values may be higher or lower depending on your calorie needs.

Figure 2

A smarter choice is to select skim milk (non-fat milk) instead. Take a look at the nutrition facts above (Figure 2), for the same serving size of skim milk. Here you can see that the carbohydrate, protein and calcium are almost exactly the same. There is a noticeable decline in the cholesterol, but take look at the total fat and saturated fat. Zero. This means that no fat will be stored from the same serving size of milk as previous. As a result, your body will shred stored body fat immediately after it burns off the glass of skim milk. It's a minor change, but a significant one. As you can see, the missing fat reduces the number of calories, which were at 146 for the whole milk.

Making this simple change also allows you to increase your serving of milk. This supplies your body with more carbohydrate, protein and calcium, but without any fat. The most important lesson to learn here is to look at the fat on nutrition labels and compare them to the size the serving. Even low-fat milk can be high in fat if you are drinking 3 or 4 servings.

Nutrition Facts	
Serving Size 1 ounce (28g)	
Amount Per Serving	
Calories 167	Calories from Fat 124
	%Daily Value
Total Fat 15g	23%
Saturated Fat 1g	6%
Trans Fat	
Cholesterol 0mg	0%
Sodium 95mg	4%
Total Carbohydrate 5g	2%
Dietary Fiber 3g	13%
Sugars 1g	
Protein 6g	
Vitamin A 0% • Vitamin C	0%
Calcium 7% • Iron	7%
*Percent Daily Values are based on a 2,000 calorie diet. Your daily values may be higher or lower depending on your calorie needs.	

Figure 3

Here is one final example (Figure 3). The nutrition facts above are for a serving of almonds. As you can see, there is a little carbohydrate and a little protein. There is also a fairly large amount of fat (15 grams), but very little saturated fat. It is safe to say that nearly all the fat is "good" fat. There is one major problem here though. Look at the serving size. 1 ounce (28g) is less than one quarter of a cup of almonds. It's barely enough to feed a child, let alone an adult. This is not a wise choice for a meal. A small snack maybe, but not a meal. If you ate an entire cup of almonds, you would have a fat intake of 60 grams. You would also be receiving very little fuel and energy from carbohydrate; thus, effecting your metabolism.

> # Eating a fat-free diet (non-fat) is always the best choice if you intend to eat more.

Food and Meal Ideas

In case you don't have any idea about where to start for meal ideas, I have provided some examples on the next page. These are just basic meal ideas and examples. You can mix them up or just use the ones that you prefer. You can even create your own, but these examples will help you decide where to start. The meals listed, each have one thing in common. They are all well-balanced with sufficient carbohydrate and protein, but contain no more than 5 grams of fat. This constitutes a fat-free diet, but remember that you will be adding essential fatty separately.

Breakfast	Lunch	Pre-workout	Dinner
- 1 bowl of bran flakes - skim milk - whey powder (protein) - 1 banana (medium)	- 1 turkey sandwich - 1 side of salad & vinegar. - 1 large apple	- plate of pasta (med.) - non-fat pasta sauce - can of tuna (mixed into pasta sauce)	- lean beef (no external fat) - steamed rice - steamed vegetables - non-fat ice cream (1 cup)

- 2 pieces of toast (multi-grain bread) with jam - 1 apple (large) - 6 egg whites	- 1 salad with vinegar. - 1 baked potato (large) - 1 side of lentils - 1 can of tuna (in water)	- 1 banana smoothie - 1 scoop whey power (20 grams of protein) - 1 fat-free cereal bar	- grilled chicken breast, bbq sauce, & vegetables - 1 dinner roll. - Fruit salad
- 1 bowl of oatmeal - skim milk - whey powder - 3 chopped strawberries	- steamed white rice - grilled chicken breast. - 1 large pineapple ring - Teriyaki sauce	- 1 raisin bagel - 1 pear (medium) - glass of skim milk - whey powder.	- lean turkey breast - baked potato - steamed vegetables - non-fat frozen yogurt(1cup)
- 2 pieces of toast (multi-grain bread) - 4 egg whites (+ ketchup) - non-fat yogurt (small tub)	- 6 inch subway sandwich (choice of chicken, turkey, ham, beef), mustard/ vinegar - apple slices	- 1 protein shake (whey powder, skim milk) - raisin bran cereal (mixed in with shake)	- 1 portion lean veal (no external fat) - sourdough bread - side of salad - black beans

- 1 bowl of Special K (cereal) - skim milk - whey powder - 1 orange (large)	- 1 toasted tomato + cheese sandwich (non-fat cheese) - 1 portion of grilled salmon - ¼ cup of raisins	- white rice - kidney beans (mixed with rice) - 1 can of tuna (water) - 1 pear (medium)	- lamb kabob (lean) grilled, with BBQ sauce - grilled vegetables (side) - french bread stick (portion controlled)

Again, these meals are just simple ideas for you to start with. Feel free to be creative and make your own meals. As long as your meals are balanced (carb to protein), portion controlled and fat-free, you will be shredding body fat after burning them off. It goes without saying that men will have slightly bigger portions of these meals, than women. There is no way of calculating exactly what size your portion will be, because everyone is different. At the beginning of the program this may be a little confusing, but with practice, it will become easier. You simply have to experiment with which portions are suitable, then concentrate on burning them off (with activity and time). Certain foods provide more energy than others, but be aware of this and use your hunger signal as a guide to eating again. This is not mathematics; this is experience and judgment.

You may decide to add a slightly larger serving of protein to your dinners. This may help your meal digest slower throughout the night, without you waking up starving. A little extra protein after a gym workout will not hurt, but just remember not to overdo it. Overeating on protein will only put a strain on your kidneys and will go to waste. Eating a total of 30-40 grams in protein at dinner, is adequate. This extra protein may also kill off the craving for anything sweet, such as a desert.

Always try to leave yourself with appropriate time to sit down and enjoy your meals. You should be able to take your time when eating, to ensure proper digestion. I understand that some days may be so busy that you barely have time to eat, but it is crucial that you do not miss meals. In circumstances that are rushed, preparing a meal ahead of time may be necessary. Even a healthy cereal/protein bar or a protein shake with a piece of fruit, would be sufficient. The most important thing is that you avoid skipping a meal and keep your metabolism working throughout the day.

On The Go

I have already mentioned that preparing your meals ahead of time will help you to achieve eating on time. Protein shakes or meal replacement shakes can be a convenient option. In circumstances where you are unable to have a meal prepared, finding a healthy sandwich bar can come to your rescue. At a sandwich bar, it can be easy to order a meal with grilled, lean meats, while having no butter or margarine on the bread. Another healthy option is sushi. The only problem I find here is that it can be difficult finding a good, lean source of protein at a Japanese/sushi restaurant. One of my all-time favorite restaurants is Subway. They provide plenty of healthy options, and you can find a restaurant on almost any corner. The furthest that you will ever be from a Subway restaurant is 5 minutes drive, and almost anyone can tell you where one is. Very convenient!

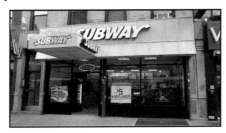

Skipping Breakfast

This is probably one of the biggest and most common of mistakes that I see among people. There is much truth behind the old saying, "breakfast is the most important meal of the day." The reason is because your breakfast is responsible for kick-starting your metabolism after 8 hours of fasting (sleeping). Skipping breakfast sends your body into shutdown and into muscle-burning mode. Bad move. Despite this, so many people ignore the importance of eating soon after they wake up in the morning. This results in irritability, drowsiness, and a lack of energy, which continues throughout the day. On top of all this, shredding body fat is brought to a complete stop.

In order to keep your body working like a fat-burning machine, which operates in tune with its metabolism, you must feed it according to the energy it consumes. This means, eating a good breakfast and eating all other meals during the day, on time. Skipping any other meals during the day, is just as bad as skipping breakfast and is a sure way to shut down your metabolism. Many people replace breakfast with a cup of coffee and maybe a piece of toast. This is not breakfast. Your body is not being provided with sufficient nutrients, therefore it will almost always have an energy crash at some stage later in the day.

One of the most important things that I want you to focus on, is to eat you meals on time. Be prepared and ready to eat when the time arrives. Plan all your meals, including your breakfast, so that there is a healthy balance of carbohydrate and protein. Each meal should provide you with a smooth energy level until your next meal. By not skipping meals, you should feel great, because your body is receiving the energy and nutrition it needs to function throughout the day. This will ensure that you keep your metabolism running constantly, so that your body continues shredding fat.

Chew Your Food

Another bit of advice that I recommend is to chew your food! What I mean by this is to avoid just shoveling down your food. Many people eat food, but they don't actually enjoy the experience until the belt around their stomach is about to break. Part of enjoying the experience of food is smelling and tasting your food. The best way to fully appreciate the taste of your food is to chew it thoroughly, before your swallow. This will also improve the digestion of the food, by reducing the work that your stomach must do to break it down.

Try this – Next time you sit down to enjoy a meal, chew every bite or spoonful 20 times. Then, swallow it. Literally, sit there for every mouthful of food and count to 20 while you chew. By the end of chewing it 20 times, the food may turn to liquid (depending on the food), but either way, it will be very well chewed and easy to swallow. Once you swallow that mouthful of food, continue to do the same thing for your next bite of food. This simple exercise will slow down the time it takes to eat a meal; making it much more enjoyable. You will notice every single bite, and completely appreciate the taste which that particular food has to offer. Even a plain piece of bread will taste great, if you take this time to enjoy every bite.

Another thing that is worthwhile mentioning is to avoid overloading your spoonfuls of food. You do not need to cram as much food as possible into your mouth, every time you eat. This doesn't mean you should take tiny bites. It means that you should take medium-sized bites, which fill your mouth comfortably. This will give you even more enjoyment from food, before you chew and swallow it. By controlling how much food you put in your mouth, each time you eat, you are controlling how long the meal will take to eat. Therefore, gaining maximum satisfaction from food.

20 Minutes To Feel Full?

There is an old theory that claims it takes 20 minutes to feel full. Apparently, this is the amount of time that it takes for the stomach to send a signal to the brain, telling you that it is full. I don't know about you, but I can eat a lot of food in 20 minutes (if I choose to). Even if I slow down my rate of eating and chew my food well, I'm sure that a regular meal would not take me 20 minutes to finish. I'm also sure that if I drink half a gallon of water in 30 seconds, I will feel sick and my brain will somehow get the message that I'm full. So, there goes the 20-minute theory out the window!

Let's be honest, the last thing that you want to be thinking about when you eat, is the clock. Meals should be about taking your time, savoring and enjoying every bite of food; then finishing! **The amount of food that you have chosen should be predetermined.** No matter what size the meal is, you should commit to it beforehand. You should already have decided on the type of food and the size of portion, which are best for your health and that particular time of day. Then, simply eat it and enjoy it. On *Shred Body Fat*, emotions do not come into play, but management does. There is no going back to the fridge for more food. If you feel that you have shortchanged yourself, learn and take a mental note for next time. This type of discipline is important.

Vegetarians

If you happen to be a vegetarian and are planning on doing the *Shred Body Fat* program, your biggest challenge will be obtaining sufficient protein from your food. It can be done, but many of the quality lean proteins come in the form of chicken, turkey, beef or fish. If you allow yourself to eat eggs and drink milk, the problem may be a little easier to solve. A great source of protein can also come from whey, but variety is an important element in this program. Many other foods which have small amounts of protein in them (such as beans, nuts, and lentils), will not have a huge impact on your protein requirements. Even soy protein is likely to leave you short of strength and stamina while on *Shred Body Fat*.

To combat the effect of excluding valuable proteins from your diet, you will have to be determined to prevail. Plan and decide exactly what foods you will allow yourself to eat and how you will get a portion containing 20-30 grams of protein, per meal. Your workouts will need to be extremely focused, just to maintain your strength. It is certainly possible to shred fat while still remaining a vegetarian or vegan, but expect limitations on the muscle and strength that you acquire. Definitely focus on muscle and strength maintenance, not gains, as you lose weight.

4. Exercise (battle plan)

Losing weight

Losing weight is fairly easy, but losing fat requires more precision. If you simply want to lose weight, there are many diets and strategies that can achieve this for you. Using these methods can help you to drop 10-15 pounds in a week just by dehydrating yourself or using diuretics. By sending your body into a ketosis state, you can drop even more weight. Bodybuilders, boxers and wrestlers do it all the time to make a weight class, but this is only ever short-term. The weight always comes back after a day or two. Putting your body through this kind of torture to achieve a brief weight-loss is unhealthy and it sets you further back from your weight-loss goal. The proper way to lose fat is by using a controlled diet which creates a slight calorie deficit, then rebuilding muscle that was lost.

The Truth about Six Pack Abs

One of the biggest misconceptions in the fitness industry is that in order to attain a six-pack (visible abdominal muscles), you need to do abdominal exercises. I am going to destroy this myth right now. Ab exercises will make your abdominal muscles bigger and stronger, but they will only have a slight effect on the appearance of them. This is because ab exercises DO NOT burn fat from your abdominal area. Your body burns fat from the last area it stored fat, and not by way of sit-ups or crunches. The reason that people struggle to lose their last couple inches of belly fat is because it is the first place that they stored it as a baby, and it has been there the longest.

Some may argue that doing ab exercises will build the muscles in that area of the body; therefore, enhancing metabolism by increasing overall muscle and the amount of fat that is burnt on a daily basis. Unfortunately, this theory has proven to be very unsuccessful. In most cases, people who train abs as a part of their gym routine (with the intent of achieving a six-pack), end up tiring themselves out with the wrong focus. They achieve minimal results and may even become disheartened when they see a larger abdominal area, rather than a smaller, ripped one.

The *Shred Body Fat* program allows you to train smarter, not harder. It is not advised to ever train abs during this program. Instead, training abs should be left until the time when you have achieved a body-fat percentage that is low enough for your abs to already be seen. Even then, ab exercises remain optional. On *Shred Body Fat*, ab training will be taken care of by other body movements. For example, when you are training chest and lifting at your maximum capability, your body will automatically be using your ab muscles to balance and support your core throughout the lift. When the weight that you are lifting is heavy enough to challenge you, your abs will benefit just as much as doing a concentrated ab exercise. Therefore, doing abs after chest, becomes redundant.

When training triceps, abs would be used secondary once again, without you even realizing. Basically, your entire mid-section must remain firm and rigid in order to complete a tricep movement at full intensity. The heavier the weight, the harder and stronger your abs must become to support your body, arms and triceps. I, myself, have proved that abs can be built to an amazing level, just by lifting with greater intensity on other body parts. My shredded six-pack was achieved in that exact way, without ever doing ab exercises. I can also do just as many sit-ups as anyone who spends hours training their abs. You too, can achieve this same abdominal strength and appearance, just by using high intensity.

The Secret to a Six-pack

Simply put, a six-pack can be achieved by shredding fat from your body, until the layer around your stomach and mid-section is minimal. This part of the body is often a problem area for most people, due to the body's natural tendency to store fat there first. The good news is that your six-pack is something that already exists. You simply require proper diet and exercise to reveal it.

Abdominal Muscles

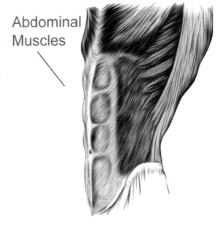

The body burns fat from the last place that it stored fat.

Therefore, abdominal fat is often the last to be removed, because it has been there the longest.

It is safe to say that you do not ever have to do a single sit-up or ab exercise, to achieve a six-pack. Ab exercises do nothing to achieve fat-loss around your abdominal area. Instead, they merely consume time and energy which could be better spent, shredding fat from your body directly. This is where you can absorb the knowledge from this book and put it to good use. It is about working smarter, not harder. When you work smarter, your body will have no choice but to burn fat as a source of energy, until the fat stores around your belly have been completely removed.

The fastest way to achieving a six-pack is to have your focus on the real problem. The real problem is the layer of fat that surrounds the abdominal area. Once this layer is gone, you may do all the sit-ups that you desire to. Only then, will the visual benefits be noticeable from doing ab exercises. As you continue to shred fat from you mid-section, you will begin to see your six-pack and realize that you actually already had one. You were simply unable to see it before. Once you see this six-pack appear, you can make the decision to enhance these muscles even further with ab exercises, or not even bother. Either way, you will have a six-pack.

Cellulite

Cellulite is a term used to describe the dimpled appearance of skin around the thighs and buttocks. It is usually more common in women than men, but varies depending on the individual. Cellulite is simply fat that has been removed from its fat cell, but is trapped by connective tissue. This gives the skin surrounding it an unsightly appearance, which can be mistaken for a skin condition. It is not a skin condition, it is a body fat condition. The good news is that this fat is easily accessible by the body, as a source of energy. Once the fat in this area of the body has been used and burnt as energy, the cellulite will no longer be there. Removing cellulite can be accomplished on the way to achieving your fat-loss goal. Don't waste your money on special creams, remedies or surgery. *Shred Body Fat* will handle it without any problem.

Your Overall Focus

The focus for shedding body fat is to MAINTAIN your strength, while you are losing body fat and dropping weight. Muscle growth is not going to be your first priority. If it was, then eating more food and calories (to gain weight, size and strength) would be implemented. I am not saying that you cannot make muscle gains when shredding body fat, but it is ideal to focus on maintaining muscle, rather than increasing it. This will still enable optimal fat-burning, without eating the excess calories which would obviously hinder your fat-loss. You can easily gain more muscle and size, once you have reached your target body fat percentage or weight (if you choose to). In fact, gaining size and muscle requires some dedication, but compared to shredding body fat, it's a piece of cake!

Getting the basic core principles right and practicing them consistently as part of your life, is the most important part of *Shred Body Fat*. Weight training is simply a tool for you to use for keeping you strong, while removing fat from your body.

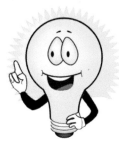

Remember, size gains always look better on a lean, shredded body. First concentrate on shredding those unwanted fat stores; then, let your muscle size follow naturally, with better definition and appearance.

The Difference Between

Men and Women

I have said previously that *Shred Body Fat* is designed for both men and women equally. This is because it is based on the scientific principles of how the human body uses fat as a source of energy. It makes no difference if you are a man or a woman. Everyone is different and everyone may lose body fat at different rates, but the principles still apply equally. Human evolution, genetics, enzymes and the fundamentals of metabolism, all remain the same for every person.

Because men and women have different energy requirements, there will be two minor differences that influence this. These are: 1) The amount of food eaten 2) The amount of weight lifted. Men will be eating slightly more calories on a daily basis, and will generally be lifting heavier weight. Aside from those two factors, the program is exactly the same for both genders. Weight sessions are based on having short workouts with YOUR maximum intensity. This means, the percentage level of your intensity should be the same as anyone else on *Shred Body Fat*. That is, 100%.

Short weight sessions, allow you to maintain your freshness and keep your intensity at its maximum. Do not become intimidated by the term "maximum intensity." It simply means that you are giving your absolute best. This applies to both men AND women. Find a weight which is not too heavy, but still heavy enough to challenge you; then "explode" into the set. This can be learned and applied by anyone. If you are a woman, and are uncomfortable with that idea, think of "explode" as simply trying your best. That's all it really means. With time, both men and women can have similar results, in regards to progress.

3 Ways To Shred

The 3 major ways that *Shred Body Fat* achieves fat-loss are:

1. Morning Cardio

2. Between Meals

3. Muscle Repair

How Much Can You Expect To Lose?

The fat that you lose from doing cardio is measured by the amount of time you spend doing it. This calculates to approximately 10 grams of fat per 20 minutes, for men; and 7.5 grams of fat per 20 minutes, for women. This only occurs after the first 20 minutes of exercise, which your body needs to start using fat as a source of energy. Therefore, a 40-minute walk, on an empty stomach, will burn 10g of fat for men and 7.5g of fat for women. Additionally, a 60-minute walk will burn 20g of fat for men, and 15g for women. If you consider yourself to be unfit, start with a 40-minute walk, three times a week. As your fitness progresses, you can increase the walk to one hour. This equates to 40 minutes of pure fat burning.

There are other ways that you will be shredding body fat on a daily basis, but 15 to 20 grams is plenty for just 1 hour of cardio. This amount of fat may not seem like much, but remember that this is real body fat. When this fat-loss is combined with the fat-loss from eating a balanced diet and muscle recovery after weight training, the results are incredible. If you feel that you are handling the early morning walks fairly well, you can always increase them to 5, 6 or 7 days per week.

Let's take a look at how the figures stack up from simply doing cardio during your mornings. If you do a 1-hour walk, three times a week, you will be burning 60g (45g for women) of fat from your body every week. Again, this may not seem like much, but let's multiply these weeks by 12 (3 months). After 12 weeks, and applying the discipline of walking three times a week, a man will have burnt 720g of fat; while a woman will have burnt 540g. This equates to 0.72kg (1.58lbs) for men, and 0.54kg (1.19lbs) for women. That's pretty impressive considering the weight that is being lost is pure fat (not muscle or water), and just by doing cardio correctly. After walking 6 days a week, for 12 weeks, men can expect to lose 3.17lbs of body fat; while women can expect to lose 2.38lbs! This is body fat that will never be seen again, because it is removed permanently.

Below is a photo of what 1 Kilogram (2.2 Pounds) of fat looks like.

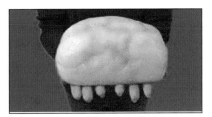

1kg of fat (2.2lbs)

Total Fat Loss on *Shred Body Fat*

Shred Body Fat aims to help you to burn between 30-50 grams of pure fat from your body, every day. For some people, this amount may be more, depending on their size, gender and metabolism. On the days that you do cardio, it is reasonable to expect a minimum of 50 grams of fat-loss per day. Like I said, this figure can be higher for some people, and may even be as high as 100g per day. You can maximize your daily average by optimizing your *Shred Body Fat* plan. Optimizing simply consists of being on-time with your meals, gym sessions, and morning walks. Be ready to meet the demands that your schedule has set for your day.

In a short space of time, your body with adapt the to demands of *Shred Body Fat*. This is because *Shred Body Fat* is designed to work with your body's natural ability to burn fat. As you move through the program, you will find that your busy, active lifestyle will give you more energy. This will be energy that you never knew you had, while your results and body transformation gives you the motivation to continue strongly.

If we increase cardio to 6 days a week, while burning 50 grams of fat on each of those days, 300 grams of fat-loss is achieved during that week. Over a 3 month period this equates to 3.6kgs (7.9 lbs) of body fat! So, on a monthly basis, you can expect to look in the mirror and see yourself minus 1.2kg (2.6lbs) of body fat. Believe me, very few people can achieve this real body fat-loss in there entire life span, let alone 1 month. This would be an amazing change to the shape of your body, which everyone (including yourself) can notice and appreciate.

Throw Out Your Scale

A lot of people use their bathroom scale as a way of assessing their results. Unfortunately, the weight measured by a scale, cannot give you a true indication of fat loss/gain and muscle loss/gain. Another problem is that the weight on a scale can change dramatically on a daily basis, depending on your water levels. This can be misleading and it may even discourage you if the weight is not the feedback that you expected. There is no way of knowing exactly how much body fat you have lost on a single day. Even if you were to lose 50g of fat on a particular day, the amount is so small that it cannot be seen missing and you would not even notice it gone. Unfortunately, most fat-measuring systems are unable to measure with the degree of accuracy that can inform you perfectly.

Your mission is to simply trust in science and the human body's fat requirements per day (40 and 60). By working with these figures, you can re-evaluate each month, simply by witnessing your results with your own eyes. To do this, I recommend that you look at your entire body in the mirror, but no more than once a month. Your focus must be on completing the program and letting the results take care of themselves. Either way, it will take at least one month to notice definite changes in the amount of fat that you carry around your body. After each month, I can personally guarantee that when you look in the mirror, the difference will be clearly noticeable. *Shred Body Fat* is not guesswork. It is a system that programs the body to use and rely on body fat as a secondary source of energy, while using food as a primary source. Therefore, results are certain. Time is the only thing that stands between you and your fat-loss goal.

Genetics

Your body style and shape depends greatly on your genetic makeup. Your genetic makeup or expression consists of genes that come from both of your parents. This combination will determine your body's natural size and state when not exposed to physical training. When lifting and weight training is added to one's lifestyle, these genes will respond in either size gain or strength gain. Sometimes there will be a combination of both. This explains the man in the gym who is incredibly strong, but without all the size and mass of a bodybuilder. It also explains the natural bodybuilder who is very big and muscular, but only moves a relatively small amount of weight for his size. Even people who are not members of the gym, can fall into the naturally muscular category or naturally strong category.

Your genetic makeup is basically the "hand of cards" that you were dealt with when you were born. This does not mean that you are unable to improve on your physical size or strength, if lacking the ability in either. It simply requires you to focus on that particular area, and make smart adjustments to your diet and training. For example: If you are naturally strong and desire to make gains in size, then you should concentrate on a higher calorie intake, muscle enhancing supplements, and weight training with more repetitions. Alternatively, if you are naturally larger and possess greater muscle, but want more strength; you should concentrate on quality of food, selection of vitamins, and shorter weight sessions. These sessions should be with high intensity and longer rest periods between workouts.

An different strategy to follow is to simply work with what you have been given and use that to your advantage. What I mean by this is if you are naturally smaller but stronger, then train to continue increasing your strength. If you are a larger, more muscular build, then continue to increase your size, shape and definition, without worrying too much about the amount that you can lift. Both directions can promote good health and confidence. It is simply up to you and what your motives are at the gym. Do you want to look like one of the strongest or actually be one of the strongest? Either way, your primary motivation should always be to increase your fitness, for the purpose of living a long, healthy life.

Weight Training

Weight (resistance) training works by causing microscopic damage and tearing to the cells of your muscles. By feeding your body with the correct diet, your muscles are forced to regenerate and grow stronger. The breakdown of muscle fibre is called Catabolism; the repair and re-growth of muscle tissue is called Anabolism. *Shred Body Fat* takes full advantage of these processes.

Your muscles are the parts of your body that are responsible for burning fat 24 hours a day. Even when you sleep, your muscles will be slowly burning fat. The more muscle that you have, the faster your metabolism will be. Therefore, you must always maintain your muscle. Weight training is the method that is used to complement the *Shred Body Fat* program. No matter what gender, age, size or shape you are, training with weights or resistance will help you to maintain and rebuild your current muscle. Because this program focuses directly on shredding fat from your body, some muscle-loss cannot be avoided. To compensate for this loss, weight training is necessary.

A day of shredding fat should consist of:

✓ Balanced diet

✓ Smart cardio

✓ Good sleep

Weight training is used to support and enhance these three things. Although you are not burning fat directly when weight training, you are keeping your metabolism at its peak performance for an entire day. This allows cardio, diet and sleep to operate at their full fat-burning potential. Essentially, it holds the 3 together and is the core of *Shred Body Fat.*

Fat Shredding Triangle

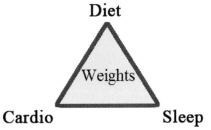

The way to know that you are not losing valuable muscle during *Shred Body Fat*, is by working hard to maintain your strength at the gym. You can do this by remembering what your numbers are on the machines and free-weights. Then, try to equal or better these at the next visit. There is no need to measure your body size or body weight. Your numbers on the machines and weights are your guide. *Shred Body Fat* is about maintaining or gaining strength, while you lose weight. It's not about the size of your muscles. Gaining muscle size can come after the program (if you choose).

Warming Up

It goes without saying that before doing any time of resistance training, you must first be completely warmed up. This is even more important when you are doing a short, high-intensity workout. In order to exercise with sufficient strength and power, your muscles must be well prepared for the moment that you actually lift the weight. This will ensure two things - 1) You get your best results, 2) You avoid any type of injury. Most people know how to warm up, but it surprises me how many people don't even bother to do it properly.

I'm going to explain exactly how to warm up, but I'm also going to keep it brief. Warming up consists of doing a preliminary movement in the exact same way as your final movement, but with a lighter weight. Anywhere from 2-4 sets is sufficient, until you feel comfortable that your muscles are warm. Make the first set very light, then gradually increase the weight, but remain well beneath the weight that you intend to give your best effort to. Remember, this is just a warm-up. You want to apply just enough energy to get warm, without taking away from your real lifts. Once you feel that you are warm and physically prepared for your best effort and heaviest weight, start to mentally focus on giving 100% to the next sets.

Stretching can also be implemented into your warm-up routine, but it is secondary. The real warm-up will come from practicing the motion of the exercise with a lighter weight. Stretching simply helps promote ligament, tendon and muscle flexibility, which can still contribute to the lift. Stretching is also beneficial in the rehabilitation of an injury, by "ironing out" tendon and ligament damage, until full recovery. This is achieved by increased blood flow (oxygen) to that particular area of the body.

My Number 1 Fat Burning Secret

Many of my clients have asked me over the years, what is the most important thing that they should do to lose weight? The answer is, there is no one, single thing. Losing body fat is purely scientific and requires the combination of many skills in order to resist your body's natural tendency to store fat for survival. It is this combination of skills that will encourage your metabolism to reverse the process of storing, and begin the process of shredding. Your determination to achieve this can be responsible for losing all the weight that you would ever want to lose.

I'm not going to lie to you and say that losing weight is easy. It is definitely a challenge. However, this book is dedicated to overcoming that challenge by giving you the tools that you need. My goal is to eliminate all the confusion associated with losing body fat and send you in the right direction. This way, reaching your goal will become inevitable.

Now you know that shredding body fat is a process and requires a combination of skills, I'm going to share with you a secret which

115

may help you the most. I always describe this as my "Number 1 Secret," but really it's just a huge weapon. There are many other weapons in this book, so apply them all. My biggest weapon (secret) is this: **Do a Chest and Back workout, once a week.** Chest and Back have proved to be tremendous in shredding body fat. They are great fat burners which continue to keep your metabolism high for days at a time. The reason for this is simply because they are both large areas of muscle, which are used frequently during daily life. You use them all the time, without even knowing. Due to their core situation, they play a big part in overall energy consumption.

Training these two body parts on separate days, once a week, will leave you with plenty of recovery time in between workouts. It will also leave your body with a constant fat-burning routine, as a result of strong muscles which are continuously being repaired. Your body will become a fat-burning furnace! A schedule of twice a week is not too demanding. It simply requires some discipline and dedication, but consistency is the key. Chest and Back have helped many of my clients transform their bodies in a relatively small amount of time, and it can do the same for you. Your results are guaranteed to amplify and your goal will be reached even faster.

Legs (another option)

Another major body part and large muscle group is Legs. Along with Chest and Back, Legs can be a major fat-burner. The thigh and hamstring area of your leg is great for fueling your metabolism. We use our legs constantly throughout the day for walking and standing. As we sleep at night, our legs also require energy to burn and repair for the next day.

Some people (myself included) do not feel the need to train their legs with weight at the gym. This is because genetically they already have strong, muscular legs or they spend a lot of time walking and being physical on their feet, outside of the gym. If you don't have strong legs and you feel the need to make them stronger with weight training, then do so. It's really a personal preference as to whether you train your legs or not, but they can definitely become a major fat-burner if you do decide to strengthen them. I would suggest that you make this decision early in your *Shred Body Fat* program, but you can certainly change your mind if you feel the need to. The more major fat-burners that you have, the better.

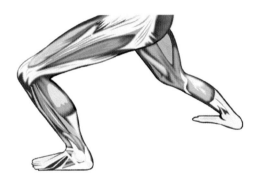

Training Minor Muscles (secondary)

Minor muscles are not considered to be major fat-burners, but they do complete your total strength and physical appearance. Try to view these muscles as additions to your workouts, and do not let them consume too much of your focus. Your focus should be reserved for the major muscles, which are responsible for burning large amounts of fat. Generally, secondary muscles are left up to the individual's preference and what he or she considers to be necessary. For example, some people want bigger, stronger forearms, so they spend more time building their forearms and wrists. Other people prefer bigger, stronger biceps, so they work on biceps instead. Women may prefer to work on their upper leg and buttock region.

It is common for some men to have naturally thin legs, so they might choose to work on their calf muscles to balance the rest of their body out. Others with naturally bigger legs, may leave them out of their workout entirely. The decision as to which minor muscles you should train, is purely a personal preference. For people who are not sure which muscles will add to their physical appearance, I suggest that you strip down naked and look at yourself in the mirror. This way, you can make a decision on two or three specific body parts which you would like to be firmer and stronger. These are the ones that will sculpt the look you want. Some popular examples are: calves, hamstrings, buttocks, biceps, forearms, wrists, triceps, rear deltoids (rear shoulder muscles), and neck muscles.

Take your pick of the two or three muscles that you prefer to focus on, and don't bother with the rest. This program is about removing fat from your body, not about making every single muscle in your body perfect and strong. Almost all your muscles get used during primary-muscle exercises anyway, so training them individually becomes unnecessary. *Shred Body Fat* requires you to focus on the major fat-burning muscles (primary muscles), and select only a few secondary muscles to complete the shape of the body that you desire. This is key. Keep it simple and remember that your number 1 goal is to reach your weight-loss target in the shortest space of time, by shredding body fat. Once you reach your goal, you can add more secondary muscles to your workout, if that's what you choose.

Lifting Weights

The choice is yours as to how you prefer to attack your weight training, but the most important thing is that you actually do implement a weight session 2-3 times a week. This will simply be a major tool for reaching your weight-loss goal faster. Keeping a consistent routine for weight training every week, will maintain your strength and muscle mass while you shred your unwanted body fat. It is also important that you keep your sessions short, but with high intensity. Concentrate on limiting your sets to a minimum, while being able to summon the strength to move a weight that challenges you the most. Another reason for the short weight sessions is to keep you from losing motivation. Nobody wants to be stuck in the gym for hours and hours. Get in, warm up, lift weight, and get out!

On the next page, there are some examples of different exercises for resistance and weight training. These are generally the most common exercises. but whichever you choose is up to you. Just remember to choose the exercise that works your targeted muscle the best, and use that exercise to get stronger by increasing the weight. Doing many different exercises for one body part will not shock the muscle more than increasing the weight resistance. This is how you will gauge that you are getting stronger. Some body parts that you may personally prefer to strengthen and tone, might not be listed below. You can research what exercises are good for those body parts, then select the one that you feel is getting the best results.

Chest

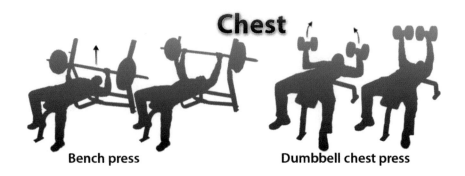

Bench press

Dumbbell chest press

Back   # Legs

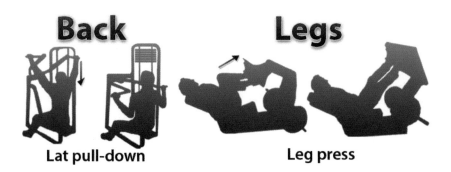

Lat pull-down   Leg press

Shoulders

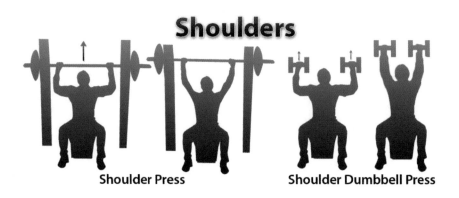

Shoulder Press   Shoulder Dumbbell Press

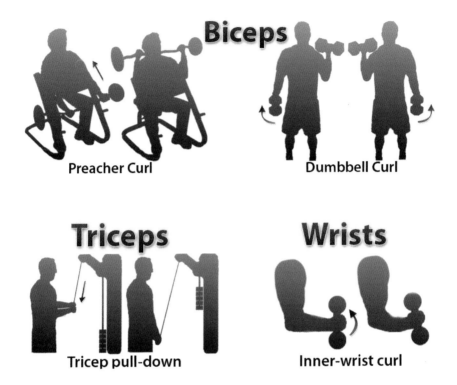

Preacher Curl   **Dumbbell Curl**

Tricep pull-down   **Inner-wrist curl**

No Gym Membership?

If you do not have a gym membership I would sternly suggest that you invest in one, at least for 3 months. The facilities in a gym make it easy to do resistance training with weights or machines. If for some reason, you cannot join a gym, there are alternatives. You could train at home by investing in a bench, some weights and barbells. Obviously, they also require space to store them in, so that may not be possible either. As a very last resort, you can use your own body weight for resistance exercise. There are numerous exercises that only require your own body weight to achieve a good muscle workout. These include: push-ups (chest, arms), squats, lunges (legs, lower back), and pull-ups (upper back, shoulders).

Note: pull-ups are great for an entire body workout, but require something to hold on to. They may also only be suited to people that have the strength to pull their own weight.

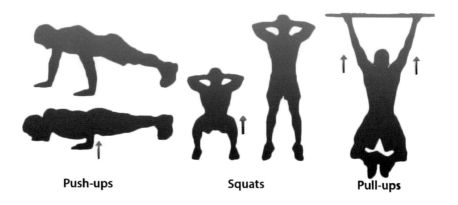

Push-ups   **Squats**   **Pull-ups**

The results that you get from these exercises may be limited and can no way compare to the increasing of weight resistance that a gym would offer. Therefore, the focus should remain entirely on maintaining your strength, not building it. You may want to increase repetitions slightly more than you would when working with machines or weights. This is because you will need to compensate for the disadvantage of not being able to increase the weight resistance and shock to your muscles. A lean body will still be achieved without the aid of a gym, provided you stay focused on your diet, morning cardio, and maintaining your strength.

"Perfect Form" – Think Again

The first thing that any personal trainer will tell you when weight training, is to focus on "perfect form." What this means is to concentrate on the technique of moving the weight, rather than concentrate on the amount of weight that you are actually moving.

In other words, focus on lifting the weight with perfect technique. This may have worked for you in the past, and over a long period of time you may have experienced decent results. That's great, but I am here to tell you that perfect form is NOT the best way to shred body fat.

"Perfect form" is a concept that derives mostly from fitness trainers and bodybuilders. It basically involves doing the technique of moving a weight in such a slow, stiff and rigid motion, so as to prove that you have complete control over the weight that you are lifting. In theory, this targets the muscle that you are training, in a more concentrated way. By targeting that muscle and only that muscle, you are encouraging better growth. With more repetitions, hypertrophy (muscle growth) is achieved.

Unfortunately, shredding body fat is an entirely different ball game. The reason "perfect form" is not suitable for shredding fat, is because that same motion includes putting a lot of unnecessary strain on your tendons, joints and ligaments; while only shocking the muscle slightly. This is because you are lifting a weight which you are too comfortable with. With a normal, high calorie diet, you may handle the strain that your tendons and ligaments suffer; when on the *Shred Body Fat* program, this strain will be too much and can lead to injury. This will become a problem. Simply put, perfect form will not encourage muscle growth at a high enough level so as to leave your joints, ligaments and tendons unaffected.

This brings us to "Relaxed Form."

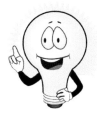

Relaxed Form

Relaxed Form is a term which describes doing a weight movement with sufficient technique, so as to hit the muscle intended. This means your form is not perfect, but it is still good enough to reach your target muscle. This way, you are not limited by striving for perfection. The last thing you want is to resemble a robot when doing strength training.

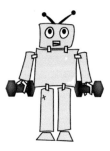

Limiting, is the best word to describe perfect form. Relaxed form, on the other hand, enables you to unleash your true strength potential. There is no evidence to suggest that lifting a slightly heavier weight in a slightly relaxed manner will increase the risk of injury. In fact, studies have shown that most injuries are a result of stiff, full-range movements, which provide no significant strength gains at all. For this reason, it makes sense to use a method of weight training which enhances your strength efficiently, while minimizing the chance of injury. **Relaxed form does not mean sloppy form.** Relaxed form means summoning your strength to lift the weight, but not obsessing over how perfectly you lift the weight. This still requires good form, but your real strength potential will become enabled.

If you are like me, you don't want to spend your entire life in a gym. Most people have busy lives and other commitments. They would rather be doing other things than trudging around at the gym, for many hours. Fast, effective results are what you should strive for. Relaxed form will give you this, by shocking your muscle with a slightly heavier weight that challenges you. Every time you introduce a new weight to your muscles, they respond by becoming stronger for the next workout. This is a winning formula for shredding body fat.

Limit Range of Motion

The term "full range of motion" is another term that is thrown around a gym by so-called experts. Unfortunately, what most people think is a full range of motion, is usually an exaggerated version of an exercise which serves little purpose. Again, this idea brainwashes people into thinking they are doing an exercise the correct way, when in fact, they are not.

There is only so much range of motion that you can use for an exercise, before you start working a different muscle than the one that you are intending to strengthen. What this means is that if you are lifting with a full range of motion, you are actually capable of lifting heavier with the muscle that you were targeting. This is because the full range forces you to lift the weight with smaller muscles, thus denying the larger muscle of its full potential. In other words, if you are capable of lifting a weight with smaller muscles, you are capable of lifting a lot more with larger ones.

Take a look at the range of motion in the two examples

on the next page.

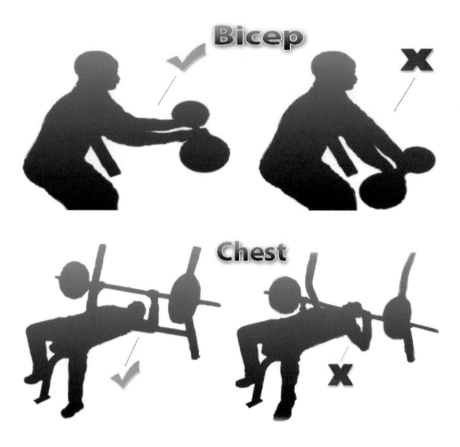

The above illustrations show the correct and incorrect ways to do these types of exercises. In both incorrect cases, smaller muscles are being forced to lift the weight, once a certain range has been met. For the Bicep Preacher Curl, forearms are used; for the Chest Bench Press, front deltoids are used. These full range movements would be fine if you were intending to strengthen forearms and front deltoids, but you are not. Plus, there are many better exercises for those particular body parts, so it's not smart either way. Your intention is to strengthen chest and biceps from the above two exercises. To do this, limit your range, and challenge yourself with a heavier weight. Once again, this will bring out your full strength potential.

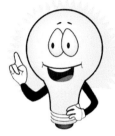

Tip: A great way to implement your weight training is to structure your workouts around "Compound Movements." Compound Movements are exercises which require you to use many muscles, within an individual exercise. For example: a Leg Press is a compound movement which requires you to use many different muscles in your leg, all at the same time. This would be a much better exercise for maintaining strength and shredding fat during the long-term, as opposed to a Leg Raise, which only targets a specific area of the leg. Compound Movements also greatly reduce the risk of an injury, due to the overall strength they bring to an entire group of muscles. This translates into faster, better results.

How Long To Rest Between Sets

Many people ask me, "how long should I rest in between sets?" I always answer with, "how ever long you need to lift with full intensity again." You may need 5-10 minutes. Even if you need more than 10 minutes, take it (but this is usually not necessary). Basically, you should have sufficient time to be physically and mentally prepared to explode into your next set. Intensity is what will enable you to overload the muscle, for best results. Obviously, you shouldn't wait too long between sets. Cooling down after a lactic acid buildup, can lead to injury. Avoid this by staying warmed up.

The purpose of not having a set limit on the time that you rest in between sets, is to be certain that you are ready for your next set. It makes no sense rushing into your next set, if you're not fully recovered from your previous set. In order to build muscle strength, you need to be improving. This means lifting better each time you lift. You cannot do this if you are not mentally and physically prepared to lift again. The shock that your muscles receive from rushing into another set is minimal, compared to the shock that they receive when ready to lift with full strength and intensity.

> **Your body needs full rest and recovery in between workouts, to achieve maximum results at the gym. It also needs full rest and recovery in between sets, to ensure maximum results from your lift.**

Challenging Yourself

You may have heard the following from trainers, acquaintances or just people who plain know-it-all: "never sacrifice range of motion, for weight!" Every time I hear this I laugh and respond with: "never limit your potential to gain strength, by being stuck on range of motion." Weight always wins over range of motion. I'll say it again, WEIGHT ALWAYS WINS OVER RANGE OF MOTION. The difference between being successful in the gym and wasting your time, is being able to unleash your true strength by challenging yourself. Challenging yourself, simply means finding a weight that you are very comfortable lifting and then lifting a little heavier. That's it. If you feel the need to reduce your range-of-motion a little, then so be it.

Every time you lift a weight that challenges you, your muscles are shocked into adjusting to that weight. Therefore, you are forced to grow stronger in between workouts. This is because your muscles are sent a signal which tells them to match the strength requirements that you were previously testing them with. This process also sends a shock to your metabolism and encourages your body to burn a greater amount of fat per day. Challenging yourself is the way that real strength is built, and is what separates different strength levels in humans. Every human conditions themself to a certain strength level, throughout the years of their life.

It is much easier to achieve results by gradually increasing weight or resistance, than forcing out as many repetitions as you can manage. This is because you are letting the weight do the work for you. Your body has no choice but to get stronger, and it will do so without the strain of countless repetitions and hours in the gym. The more repetitions and time you spend in the gym, the higher the risk of injury. Remember, you can always prove to yourself that you can easily lift a lighter weight with perfect form, but this is unnecessary. Seeing the results and gains that you make from testing yourself with heavier weight, will be enough proof.

The 4-6-8 Rule

It is a highly effective strategy to keep your repetitions at 4-6 reps. Even though you are not trying to become a power-lifting champion, you should strive to maintain your own personal strength. Whether you are bench pressing 500 pounds or 15 pounds, you must always challenge what you are capable of lifting. Keeping your workouts short, but with high intensity, ensures that you gain the most strength from of your workouts, without burning yourself out in the long run. In different parts of this book, I stress that you should not be spending hours and hours in the gym. Your focus should be about getting to the gym, challenging yourself, and then getting out. The amount of weight that you lift is what determines your results; the hours that you spend in the gym and the number of sets or repetitions that you do, does not.

The 4-6-8 rule is an excellent guide for you to use, while doing your resistance workout. It represents the number of repetitions that you can do at a certain weight and what your thoughts should be.

> 4 = The weight is a challenge and I am building strength.
>
> 6 = I am comfortable with the weight and have gotten stronger.
>
> 8 = My strength now requires an increase in weight resistance.

As you can see, it's a very simple guide that shows you when to lift heavier. Your goal is to slowly climb and increase your strength by using the repetitions as your guide. So, 4 is the number which determines that a weight is challenging you. 6 determines that you are gaining mastery over that weight. 8 grants you permission to increase the weight or resistance slightly. This increase should put you back to 4 again, and so on. Whenever you reach 8 repetitions, you should feel enough confidence in your strength to increase the weight. Through this type of patient training (along with correct nutrition), your strength will increase naturally, without struggle and pain. This is what will assist you in shredding fat perfectly.

Less is More

It is important to realize that spending too many hours at the gym is counter-productive. The more reps (number of repetitions in an exercise) that you do, the more ability you waste. This is the ability to increase the weight or resistance, allowing your fitness to advance. The more sets (number of times an exercise is done) that you do, the harder it becomes to recover for your next workout. This recovery includes physical and mental recovery. If you don't feel like going to the gym, that's an indication that you haven't fully recovered (physically or mentally) from the last workout.

I have made references throughout this book about your resistance workout sessions being short and intense. You want to have the stamina to stay on *Shred Body Fat* for as long as possible. You will give yourself every chance of doing this by working smart. I have already covered a smart strategy for the number of reps that you should do in a set. Now, for the number of sets.

Number of Sets

I advise that you keep the number of sets to a maximum of 3 sets. This enables you to have full intensity for the entire time. Remember, high intensity is what will help you to achieve your best results, in the least amount of time. Often, you will find that your second set is your most powerful and explosive. It is when your energy and strength climaxes. The third set then becomes a bonus set. You should aim to be exhausted from the first 2 sets, enabling you to use the third set as a finisher. Some people would call this third set a "super set" or "double set," but not so. You will still be giving it the same time, preparation and effort as the previous sets, to make sure it is done to the best of your ability.

Set	Intensity	Result
1st set	100%	90%
2nd set	100%	100%
3rd set	100%	70%

By the end of any exercise, you will have shocked the muscle with maximum intensity and weight, but still avoided the wear and tear that comes with long-duration training. This whole concept of "less is more" can be applied even further. My own personal workouts contain 2 sets, not 3 sets. This is because I feel like I no longer need the third set to polish my exercises. I have no problem maintaining my strength, and 2 sets makes my gym sessions even shorter. I have even read that some modern fitness trainers advocate doing only 1 set! (after having warmed up) Although this may be a little extreme, it shows that there is valid cause for shocking your muscle with intensity and weight, not volume and duration. Sets and reps should always be kept to a minimum for getting the job done.

I advise you to start at 3 sets, because this is still a tremendous change from the long, strenuous workouts that most people are used to. As you progress and find it easier to maintain your strength, 2 sets on a weekly basis (per exercise), may be applied. The important thing is that you maintain or build strength, without the mental torture and physical damage that long gym sessions will force upon you. By applying the "less is more" strategy, you will increase your muscle strength while also keeping your bone, ligament and tendon strength. Preserving your bone, ligament and tendon strength will easily transcend the results that other people produce from spending hours in the gym.

Even 3 sets goes against the advice that a lot of personal trainers will give. Unfortunately, these trainers are not thinking about your long-term results and fat-loss. I am. You want to ask yourself this question every time you walk into a gym. Will this workout build on my strength, but still give me the energy to come back to the gym in 2 days time? If the answer is yes, your workout will be appropriate. Further more, will I be able to acquire the motivation to do this 3 times per week for however long I choose? Again, your answer should be yes. Your workout should not be a chore. It should be fun and give you great satisfaction, simply because it works so well.

Rest

Your muscles do not grow when you are actually lifting weight at the gym. They grow in the days to follow, with rest and food. When shredding body fat, you have the disadvantage of not being able to feed your body and muscles excess amounts of food during recovery. This is because the focus is on creating a slight calorie deficit. Naturally, a calorie deficit can hinder muscle recovery, but you can overcome this. The way to overcome this is by being on time with your meals and training correctly.

On the *Shred Body Fat* program, you will be doing a resistance workout on three days out of every week. Even two days is sufficient, but I recommend three days for working more body parts, and creating a more balanced schedule. However, training more than three days per week is counterproductive. Do not do that. Rest is very important for your muscles on this program, because of the style of training involved, i.e. short, high-intensity workouts with muscle overload. Rest also ensures that you are fresh for your return to the gym and ready to lift as heavy or heavier than your previous session.

A three-day per week weight schedule could look like this.

Monday	Legs +Shoulders
Tuesday	(rest)
Wednesday	Back + Biceps
Thursday	(rest)
Friday	Chest + Triceps
Saturday	(rest)
Sunday	(rest)

The above is a basic plan that I have found to work well for most people, for the scheduling of weight training. Every individual is different, but I encourage you to do Chest, Back, and Legs as primary fat-burning body parts, on separate days. Secondary body parts are Triceps, Biceps and Shoulders. I specifically paired Back and Biceps together, because they are generally both pulling movements. Also, Chest with Triceps are paired together, because they are mostly pushing movements. This doesn't really apply to the Shoulders and Legs day (because they are entirely different areas of the body), but still both mainly pushing movements.

Now, the reason I described the above schedule as just a basic plan is because other minor body parts may be incorporated (depending on the individual). Those six are the most common and popular parts that the majority of people are inclined to focus on, but if you have a different preference, one can easily be replaced. For example, if you feel that your legs are already quite muscular, you may prefer to replace them with a Forearm or Wrist workout. This is fine. As mentioned previously, some people simply do not need to do legs.

If you choose to do all of the body parts that I have chosen, plus other smaller body parts such as forearms or wrists, then add them to your workouts on one of those particular days. Do not come back into the gym on a rest day. Your rest days need to be completely free of lifting anything at all, regardless of whether it is with a different body part. This rest is not only for restoring the muscles that you have trained previously, but also for restoring your heart, kidneys, liver, brain, and any other major organs in your body. The restoration of your organs is not only vital to your health, but also provides you with complete power and strength for your next workout. **Proper rest (mentally and physically) is the most important factor in achieving your very best performance at the gym.**

Muscle Memory

While you are shredding fat from your body, a reduction in the size of your muscles may occur. Do not confuse this with a reduction in muscle strength, because the two are very different things. Muscle size will usually equate to more strength, but not in all cases. This is what separates the Bodybuilder from the Strength Trainer.

I, myself, am 3 times stronger than I was 2 years ago but I am also pretty much the same size. This means that despite looking almost the same size, I lift 3 times the amount that I used to lift and my muscles are 3 times stronger, harder and denser. This is REAL muscle growth. This type of muscle growth is much longer lasting, because it is real strength that doesn't decrease rapidly like the size and muscle that bodybuilders create. Bodybuilders train themselves to create a "balloon effect" or "blow-up doll" effect for competition, with the aid of supplements, creatine and even steroids. This is not real muscle growth. Real muscle growth and strength is something that your body retains for many years to come.

The term for this long-term strength is "Muscle Memory." Muscle memory is what your muscles retain from a certain period in your life, when you were able to achieve a certain strength. Once you have this strength, your muscles can remember it for years to come. This means that even after a complete absence of training and working out, for a period of years, your body is still capable of reclaiming that strength relatively quickly. Much quicker than the original time it took to acquire. Your body simply does not have to work as hard to reach that level of strength again. For that reason, it is a wonderful thing. Just remember though, muscle memory can only be achieved through real strength gains, not size gains.

Will I look bulky if I start lifting heavier?

This seems to be a concern for most women. Men who prefer a lean, toned physique (over a bulky, muscular one), also have this concern. Many people avoid lifting a heavier weight which challenges them, in fear of becoming too muscular (such as a bodybuilder). When I first start teaching clients, I will often get the following response, "but I don't want to look a bodybuilder!" This is a common idea that belongs to many inexperienced members of the gym. It's another myth that I will now clearly dispel.

You will NOT put on size and look like a bodybuilder, simply by lifting a heavier weight. Putting on noticeable muscle size and weight is not possible through heavy lifting alone. Even if you lift heavy, then go home and eat the entire fridge, you will still struggle to look like a bodybuilder. If you eat the fridge every day for a month, you might start to look a little bulky! Aside from doing that, you will continue to look perfectly normal.

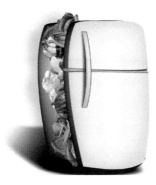

It's safe to say that you do not intend on eating the entire fridge after your workouts. In fact, the *Shred Body Fat* program is based on a slight calorie deficit, which means your chances of bulking up are zero. By using resistance training to challenge your strength potential, you will only be creating stronger, firmer and denser muscles. Bodybuilders train for hours on a daily basis (as well as feed their bodies constantly with food, creatine and other supplements) to induce size and mass. Not to mention their use of anabolic steroids to enhance testosterone and growth hormone. This leaves the rest of us, especially women, with no chance of gaining size.

If you feel a little bigger on the day after an intense weight session, I can guarantee that this will be short lived. The swelling that may occur from muscle stimulation is always temporary and may be enhanced by overfeeding during post-workout. This swelling can be minimized by a controlled food intake. It can also be used to your advantage, which is to burn fat continuously until your muscles fully recover.

Your Mental Focus

Where is your focus when you are at the gym, before the very moment that you are about to lift a weight? Are you thinking about something else or somewhere else? Are you thinking that the weight you are about to lift is going to be difficult? Or are you just thinking about how you simply do not want to be there? These are all energy consuming thoughts that will make your life difficult while moving towards your weight-loss goal.

Instead, you should be thinking about how you are going to put 100% into your next set. You only have one shot to make it count, but you are going to give it your very best effort and your highest intensity level. The thoughts you carry prior to the moment that you are about to lift are crucial and they will affect your long-term success. At the very least, you want to be thinking neutral thoughts until the seconds leading up to your lift. Then, explode!

If you think about it, your entire weight session only lasts a couple of minutes. The time that you are actually lifting only takes 10 to 20 seconds (per set), and you are only doing a few sets in total. The rest of the time in the gym should be spent relaxing, focusing and gathering your energy for the next set. You can kill some of this time by listening to music or just patiently waiting, but you must guard against negative thoughts. Once you master this routine, your weight sessions will be short, intense and painless. This is the *Shred Body Fat* way, and results will show.

Bulking up

This was a chapter that I was considering to leave out of the book, but it happens to be an important one to understand. The emphasis of this book is placed on losing real body weight, i.e. shredding body fat. So what does bulking up have to do with it?

Well, it doesn't really have anything to do with it, besides understanding how foods perform and what their role is when increasing muscle size or strength.

When striving for muscle gains, a common belief which most bodybuilders and fitness trainers have, is to simply increase protein intake. This is a mistake. Eating high levels of protein is unhealthy and puts the body under plenty of stress. It also means that your carbohydrate intake will be lower, because you can only eat so much food in a day. This creates an imbalance in the way that your body operates, because protein is not the human body's preferred source of fuel. Protein takes time to break down and only so much of it can be used at one time. Any excess protein will go to waste. Unfortunately, this is contrary to what most people think.

Sure, protein is used for repairing muscle, but eating too much of it will not provide extra muscle growth or strength. Carbohydrate is the real food that the body uses to build and strengthen muscles. Unlike protein, excess carbohydrate WILL be used by the body and will encourage muscle growth. This is especially true when combined with weight training or high physical activity. If you are planning to "bulk up," I recommend that you increase your carbohydrate intake, in order to support a heavier resistance training program. The carb increase will compensate for those extra calories burnt, and encourage real muscle growth. Whether you are bulking up or shredding down, carbohydrate will always be your primary source of energy, while proteins and fats will remain your secondary.

Work Smarter, Not Harder

Nothing describes the strategy of *Shred Body Fat* better than "work smarter, not harder." This very strategy (combined with patience and time) will ensure your success. You cannot fail on this diet and exercise program, provided you follow the steps correctly. Your results are guaranteed. You will burn pure body fat, one gram at a time, until you have reached your desired body weight. This is scientifically proven and it cannot let you down.

Now, let's get back to this strategy (or concept) of working smarter, not harder. So many people are influenced by the misconception that anything in life requires tremendous hard work, pain and suffering. The fact is, most things do not. Shredding body fat certainly falls under that category of things that do not. It may take a week or so to fully incorporate *Shred Body Fat* into your lifestyle, but the key word here is lifestyle. *Shred Body Fat* is designed so that it easily fits into any lifestyle. It allows you to go about your normal life and let the shredding take care of itself.

Now, the working smarter has to do with doing things in the correct manner, so that all the hard work is removed. I am not saying that you should cut corners or that this will be completely easy. I am saying that with a little planning, focus and determination, any crazy, hard work will be unnecessary. This is because you are using science and real evidence (not fad diets) to cut corners, without actually cutting corners. It's a direct path towards fat-loss and sculpting the body that you want.

On the next page, there is a list of things that are part of

the *Shred Body Fat* motto,

"Work Smarter, Not Harder"

The What	The How
☆ Burn 15-20 grams of fat directly, each day, without interrupting your metabolism.	➜ Direct fat-loss will be achieved by walking or slow cardio, for 40-60 minutes in the morning.
☆ Eat on time and avoid "starvation mode." This keeps you constantly burning energy.	➜ Prepare your meals ahead of time and allocate time to eat throughout the day.
☆ Leave boredom and food cravings behind. Respond only to hunger signals, when it is time to feed your body.	➜ Eat decent portions and stay busy. Instead of starving the body of calories, you will be feeding and burning them off.
☆ Completely avoid fat storage, while still feeding your body the essential fats that it needs for healthy functioning.	➜ Remove all fat from your meals by eating a fat-free diet, then add good fats separately through supplementation.
☆ Keep your energy levels and metabolism high throughout the day, with proper rest.	➜ Prepare yourself for 8 hours of sleep each night, and wake up at the same time everyday.

☆ Boost your metabolism by eating the correct macro-nutrients in the correct ratio.	→ Use carbs primarily, as the bulk of meals; use protein secondary, to balance meals.
☆ Keep your metabolism fast and working at its peak for 24 hours a day, 7 days a week.	→ Burn food and fat through daily activity, then replace muscle with resistance training.
☆ Get the very best out of your time spent at the gym and continue to increase your muscle and strength gains.	→ Keep your gym sessions short and explosive. This translates to maximum strength gains, with a minimum time spent.

Final Word on Lifting

As you continue shredding body fat, the stress and discomfort on your body may increase, no matter how perfect your form is or how much time you spend in the gym. In fact, the more perfect your form is, the more likely you are to injure yourself; likewise, the more time that you spend in the gym, the more likely you are to injure yourself. Basically, perfect form and full-ranges of motion will encourage injury, which is the very thing that they are supposed to prevent. In all my years of studying, teaching, and training, I have not seen one example of perfect form or full-range achieving great results. However, I've seen many injuries occur from them.

Your main goal in the gym is to maintain and strengthen your muscles, so as to boost your metabolism. To do this I advise that you keep your weight sessions short, strong and intense with minimum wear and tear on the parts of your body which are not muscle. Remember, you do not need to spend hours and hours in the gym. Less is more. You must work smarter, not harder. By limiting your number of sets, reps and range of motion, you will be challenging yourself with slightly heavier weight. This is the most effective way to maintain your strength.

5. Motivation (staying on track)

What Results to Expect

The purpose of *Shred Body Fat* is to provide you with the knowledge to take control of your physical health and appearance. This will teach you how to create a balanced diet and exercise program, which you can sustain for life. After 4 weeks, you will notice a change in your body. After 8 weeks you will notice a HUGE change in your body, and so will everyone else. After 12 weeks, you will feel like a completely different person, with the exact body shape that you were aiming for. The initial few days of discipline may be difficult to get used to, but once you commit yourself, it will become easier.

After 12 full weeks, when you have reached your weight-loss goal, achieving maintenance is much more simple. It simply requires you to maintain certain basic habits which ensure that you don't put the weight back on. Remember, once the fat is gone, it is gone forever! Provided you do not store it all over again. Real fat-loss is not the same as losing water or muscle. Water and muscle weight can be like a yo-yo (up and down). Real fat-loss is permanent. The only way to gain that fat back is to eat a careless diet, or gradually store it again over time. This can be avoided by the application of basic knowledge, which has been presented in this book.

Metabolism

The biggest component that affects fat-loss is your metabolism. It is easy to make the mistake of focusing on fat-loss, rather than focusing on what causes fat-loss. Your metabolism is the engine that commands your fat-loss and it needs to be switched on, everyday. Think of a car. In order for a car to burn fuel, it needs to be switched on with a key to the ignition. Food is your key to the ignition of your body. Even more precisely, carbohydrate is the correct key. Your success in losing weight and burning actual body fat will be determined by your proficiency and timing of your meals. It is imperative that your meals are on time, to get the absolute most out of your metabolism. You metabolism is your ally. Do not kill it.

Your Basal Metabolic Rate (BMR) is the number of calories that your body burns at rest, without the addition of exercise. Even when you sleep, your body has many operations in progress, which consume energy. These include blood circulation, food digestion, body temperature, cell repair, and other functions carried out by organs in the body, 24 hours a day.

Factors that contribute to your metabolism are:

◆ Age – Metabolism gradually slows down as you get older.

◆ Gender – Men generally have a slightly faster metabolism due do their extra size and strength.

◆ Weight – The heavier you are, the more energy that your body will consume everyday to move you around.

◆ Muscle Mass – The more muscle that you carry, the more furnaces you have to burn energy 24/7

◆ Height – Taller people tend to have bigger limbs and bones, which are heavier and consume more energy naturally.

Many of these may be out of your control, but the *Shred Body Fat* program is designed to transcend these. Any metabolic disadvantage that you may have, can be left behind with planning, discipline and precision. There is no such thing as a slow metabolism on *Shred Body Fat*, because you are working with your body and science. You may have noticed that next to the above heading called "Weight," I mentioned that the heavier you are, the more energy your body will consume. This can work to your advantage when starting the *Shred Body Fat* program. As time passes and you lose weight (fat), you should aim to replace it with muscle.

The Worst Thing You Can Do

To Your Metabolism

There is one thing that many people get into the habit of doing everyday, which kills their metabolism and affects their energy levels for the entire day. This one thing is, *missing breakfast*. **Do not do this.** Always give yourself some time to sit down and fuel your body with a balanced breakfast. Without breakfast, your metabolism will not start, and it will remain slow for the rest of the day. Even if you are in an extreme rush, still try to grab something quick on your way out, such as a piece of fruit and some toast. This would not be considered balanced, but at least your body will have some carbohydrate and fuel to work with after a night of fasting (sleeping). Your lunch should then contain more balance, to make up for the rushed breakfast. Overall, when shredding body fat, preparation and structure will avoid rushing or missing meals.

Caffeine

Caffeine is a drug which was legalized so many years ago, that it is now a regular part of most people's lives. Caffeine has a powerful effect on the central nervous system, which results in giving you a brief supply of energy. Eventually, the body becomes numb to this effect. It then requires more caffeine to trigger the original effect, or some caffeine to just feel normal again after withdrawal symptoms. These withdrawal symptoms may include headaches and tiredness. Anytime that you borrow energy from an unnatural source such as caffeine, you will have to pay it back at some stage. This can really throw your day out of place.

A bad habit that people acquire is having a cup of coffee as a replacement for their breakfast. By using the energy that coffee provides (in the form of caffeine) to get their day started, they are tricking their body into feeling good and having energy. Big mistake. Not only does your brain and nerves have to carry the stress of this fake energy, but the absence of carbohydrate will result in your body using muscle as fuel to burn. This means that your metabolism will not start working either. If you absolutely cannot start your day without your morning coffee, make sure that you have a complete and balanced breakfast with it. This will supply your body with the food it needs to function properly, regardless of the effect from caffeine.

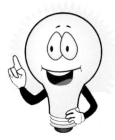

Handy tip: *Caffeine can take up to a few days to be removed from your body, through detoxification. So, if you plan to drop the habit, make sure to be patient and battle it out. After 2-3 days, withdrawal symptoms will disappear and your head will feel much clearer. This can be a good long-term investment for your energy levels. Drinking tea is another alternative. It has considerably less caffeine and even provides some healthy anti-oxidants, when taken in moderation. Ether way, the best way to achieve maximum energy, is through proper nutrition and good sleep.*

Time and Patience

Have faith in the techniques and principles until you see your body transform slowly over time. With time and patience your results will become exponential. It is simply a matter of reprogramming your body to shred fat, which doesn't happen overnight. Save yourself the time and money of fat testing or trying to measure your results. Just concentrate on the job at hand, which is to shred fat. Your results will be easily noticeable when an assessment of yourself is done on a monthly basis. You may even notice that your clothes become loose, which is another sign that you are losing weight. Many people give up on their weight-loss goal because they do not wait long enough to see the results. Do not be one of these people. The simple ideas and techniques in this book will get you to your goal, provided you are patient and allow for time.

When To Expect Results

The reason that time and patience are so important is because fat-loss is a long and precise operation. Fat stores provide more energy than carbohydrate and they burn very slowly. They are also required for use much less frequently by the body. Earlier in this book I gave you some figures to work with, in terms of fat-loss per day. These figures accumulate quite quickly over the period of a month. This is the reason I allow you to step back and take a closer look at your results, on a month-to-month basis. So, the answer to the question, "when can I expect results?" is, after one month. After 3 months, you will have an entirely new body delivered.

> **The longer that you stay on *Shred Body Fat*, the more fat you will lose.**

How Much Fat Can I Lose?

Do do not bother with body fat percentages or numbers too much. This is because they become a distraction from what is required to achieve your fat-loss goal. Numbers and figures really do not matter, provided you are happy with your body's transformation. Looking in the mirror once a month should be sufficient feedback and a good indication of your results. However, you should know the absolute minimum body fat percentage that is considered safe for men and women to have. For men it is 3% body fat and for women it is 8%. *Shred Body Fat* can easily get you to these levels if you desire, but falling below them can put you in serious danger.

An average and safer level of body fat is 8-15% for men, and 15-23% for women. Becoming shredded usually starts to occur when you get down to single digits. Most women do not necessarily want to be shredded, so achieving the firm, toned body that they want, happens around 15-20%. Dropping below this range can affect their menstrual and reproductive function. Women are genetically programmed to require more body fat than men, in order to assist their ability to have children and healthy pregnancies. Both men and women can expect fat increase and muscle decrease as they age, due to a declining metabolism.

It is important for you to know that the body needs to carry some fat to function properly. These are structural fats (not to be confused with storage fats or essential fats). Fat is used to line the walls of cells in the body, so that the cell and its membrane are protected from the outside world. Fat is also continuously required as a secondary source of fuel, in between meals. When the body cannot obtain fat for fuel, it turns to breaking down muscle tissue and organ tissue within your body. Therefore, it is rare but extremely unsafe to have a zero body fat percentage.

Structure

Structure is about ensuring that you know what your next move is going to be. It involves being prepared and having a definite plan. Once you become accustomed to the *Shred Body Fat* program, it will become natural to take the next step and make it a part of the way you live your life. *Shred body Fat* is designed to fit into your life, not interfere with it. Most people will not have any trouble implementing 4 meals into their day, but make not mistake, you must have some structure to do this.

If you can structure *Shred Body Fat* so that you are hungry straight after a gym workout, your muscles will gain an anabolic boost from the food that you then eat. In effect, you are encouraging your muscles to grow and your metabolism to remain at its peak, simply by feeding your body immediately after the workout. Your heart rate is higher than normal, and blood is still flowing to your muscles. So, carbohydrate will naturally flow to the parts of the body that were used during exercise. After 15-30 minutes, your "muscle pump" will go down and you will miss this opportunity for growth. Balancing this with eating only when you are hungry might take some practice, but is great for shredding fat. People who have so called "fast metabolisms," are usually just very good at doing this one thing. They structure their eating habits so that they eat a lot of food and burn a lot of energy, before it is time for their next meal. It is no mystery.

When using *Shred Body Fat*, try to place your attention on having structure and timing. Your structure should consist of 4 meals per day, with 3 gym sessions per week in accordance to those meals. You should always be ready for your meals, and have them prepared for when the time comes to eat. You should commit to 3-6 days per week of 40-60 minute sessions of morning cardio. This will require a little preparation the night before, so that you are ready to just walk out the door as soon as you wake up.

> **As long as you are always one step ahead, you will always have structure. This is one of the secrets to succeeding at shredding body fat.**

Optimizing Your Plan

I have already spoke briefly about optimizing your *Shred Body Fat* plan, but I want to reiterate it here. Optimizing your program simply means focusing on the key points and being on time with them. I cannot stress how important is to be on time. At the beginning, this might be difficult, because you are adjusting to the new habits. As you get used to living a *Shred Body Fat* lifestyle, those same habits will become easy. This means that your daily actions will become automatic. When this occurs, your body will apply *Shred Body Fat* 24 hours per day.

Optimizing your *Shred Body Fat* plan ensures that you burn fat all day and all night, while still feeling great and energized. Much of the feeling great part depends on how well you slept the night before. If you are not on-time with your meals, gym sessions and morning walks, your sleep curfew will be disrupted. This means that you will receive less sleep and it will affect your performance for the next day. In turn, this will cause your metabolism to slow down and you will feel fatigued and run-down.

Below are some examples of how to optimize your *Shred Body Fat* plan. Some you may do automatically, but others you may need to work on.

- Prepare your meals ahead of time

- Start morning cardio immediately after you wake up

- Keep your gym sessions brief

- Stock healthy food options at home

- Stay active throughout the day

- Prepare for sleep ahead of time by relaxing

When To Stop Shredding Fat

You will reach a point where you ultimately decide that you don't need lose anymore fat. This is the ultimate goal, but it has to be your decision. Calculating your perfect body weight has nothing to do with the number that is on the scale, or the number that is your body-fat percentage. It has to do with looking in the mirror and being satisfied with what you see. Most people are not blinded to what they want their body to look like. Once their desired look arrives, they can identify it instantly.

There are rare situations such as eating disorders, when a person's perception of their body size and image is morphed. As a consequence, they cannot make a sound judgment about their current body weight. In cases such as psychological disorders and eating disorders, it is actually possible to control unhealthy behavior with a balanced eating program and professional help. The easier that a program is to fit into your life, the less likely that these outside problems will occur. However, psychological disorders that involve eating and food, are almost always a completely separate entity to a person who has a normal goal of losing weight.

Food Sensitivity Tests

Allergy or Food Sensitivity testing may also be known as IgG ELISA Food Tests. This test is taken from a sample of blood and can produce a panel of 96 or 184, depending on how complete you want the list of foods to be. The results can benefit people in many ways, by making them aware of which foods may be responsible for negative reactions to their body. Eliminating one or two of the foods that prove to cause an effect, can make a noticeable difference to how you feel. Often, a certain food that you are sensitive to, may be replaced easily and will no longer affect your body. Many books have been written in recent times, on the subject of food sensitivity testing and the effect it has on weight control.

Unfortunately, eliminating foods that you have been tested for sensitivity towards, is not the answer to shredding body fat. Firstly, a sensitivity test can only be so accurate. The real evidence should come from your own judgment. You can achieve this by experimentation and avoiding the food that is affecting you. Then, by judging how you feel as a result, you can make a sound decision. This is called, listening to your body. Hunger signals also manifest by listening to your body. Secondly, a sensitivity towards a particular food may be the cause of several pounds of water retention and bloating. Preventing this may make you feel better about yourself when you look in the mirror, but it has nothing to do with fat-loss. If it is the bloating that you are concerned about, then go ahead and limit the food that is causing it. As far as fat-loss is concerned, ignore quick fixes and concentrate on shredding real body fat.

> Just like sit-ups, an Elisa test may be
> something to think about after you
> have reached your desired fat-loss goal.

Water Retention

Avoiding water retention has no advantage gain when trying to achieve fat-loss. If anything, dropping water weight is detrimental for 2 reasons.

1) Loosing a few pounds in water weight will slightly slow your metabolism, due to becoming lighter. Hence, there is less energy required to move your body around throughout the day.

2) Resistance workouts will suddenly become much more difficult, because you do not have the usual water weight that supports your body while lifting weight.

A much more effective way to stop bloating and water retention, is to do it slowly in congruence to the fat-loss that you achieve. This will happen on the *Shred Body Fat* program, regardless of what food you eat. The combination of a healthy, high-fiber diet and drinking plenty of water, will give your body no option but to lose more weight than the sum of the fat-loss you achieve. You may find that after dropping a pound of real body fat in a month, the scale tells you that you have lost up to 10 pounds! Much of this will be water weight and toxins that have been flushed from your intestines, so you cannot expect to lose that again in the next month.

Shred Body Fat is not only a fat-loss answer, but an entire body makeover answer. By removing fat from your body and system, you also remove toxins and food buildup within your intestines. This initial large drop in weight may be satisfying, but keep your focus on shredding body fat. Concentrate on retaining your strength at the gym, while you continue to lose weight. Ideally, muscle should replace those areas where fat was previously stored, turning you into a fat burning machine.

Staying Busy

Previously in this book, I have mentioned that in between meals you must stay busy and occupy yourself with life. I understand that this can be a challenge for many people, especially when eating food presents a great source of satisfaction in their lives. The beauty of the *Shred Body Fat* program is that it focuses on avoiding food deprivation. This can be a major cause in feeling boredom and discomfort, when changing your usual eating habits.

What must be understood is that as you move out of your comfort zone and acquire new habits that do not drain you of your energy, your life will unfold for the better. If you persist with the new habits and ideas that are presented in this book, within two weeks you will notice the difference in how you feel. Staying busy is a habit that will occur naturally, provided you can see results. After the first month is over, those results will be clearly visible and they will empower you to continue in that direction.

Be aware that the first couple of weeks may require you to manually stay busy. You may find that you have plenty of spare time and you are just waiting around for your new, shredded body to arrive. This is the best time to create new hobbies and stay busy. Staying busy can be as simple as doing laundry or walking the dog.

Below is a list of basic things to do if you catch yourself bored or thinking about food:

✔ Read a book or newspaper

✔ Walk the dog

✔ Clean your apartment/house

✔ Play a new video game or app

✔ Do grocery shopping

✔ Start a hobby

✔ Meditate

✔ Do a crossword puzzle

✔ Catch up on work

✔ Do some laundry

✔ Run Errands

✔ Surf the internet

✔ Call a friend (but avoid meeting for food)

Most people will not have to worry about boredom or killing time. *Shred Body Fat* is designed so that it fits into your normal lifestyle easily and leaves little time for boredom. The examples above are simply ideas to use if you do find that you are struggling to pass time. Again, this circumstance is highly unlikely without the deprivation of food, but the topic should still be addressed. Any time you make a change in diet and lifestyle, you are moving into foreign territory. My job is to make this transition as easy as possible and cover all your contingencies.

Obviously, there are countless other options for occupying time, depending on your interests or preferences, but the lesson here is most important. The lesson being that whenever you catch yourself thinking about food at times you are certain you are not hungry, you must get into the habit of distracting yourself. Once this habit is formed, it will always be there. You will no longer have to consciously tell yourself to go do something to occupy the few hours between meals. It will simply be automatic, and it will be part of your life. This good habit is certainly not difficult to acquire (you may already have it), but being aware of it in the beginning stages of shredding fat is definitely advantageous.

Summary

This section of the book is solely devoted to helping you remember the absolute key points of shredding body fat. They are the essentials and must be ingrained into your subconscious mind, so that you never stray from the fundamentals. If I could put this entire book into just a few lines, here is where you will find them. Anytime you are not sure of how to shred body fat, simply refer back to this section.

- **Always try to eat only when you are hungry.** This encourages a calorie deficit and makes sure that you burn a little fat from your body, after completely burning off your last meal.

- **Do not skip meals.** When you are hungry, your body needs to be fed immediately. This keeps your metabolism working and prevents it from crashing. It will also keep your day and schedule on time.

- **Additional carbohydrate or protein will not be converted to fat.** On a fat-free diet, excess carbohydrate will promote muscle and strength gain, while excess protein will go to waste. If logistics prevent you from eating when you are hungry, do not worry about weight gain. Simply accept this as extra food for your muscles, then continue on until you're hungry again.

- **Aim to do 40-60 minutes of medium-paced cardio, three times a week.** It takes 20 minutes of medium-paced cardio, on an empty stomach, before you start to directly shred fat. You can shred fat just by controlling your diet and eating only when you are hungry, but adding cardio to your mornings will boost your metabolism and kick-start your fat-shredding day.

- **Always try to increase or maintain muscle.** Muscle is the key to your consistent fat-loss. Keep a regular resistance training schedule, and avoid missing sessions. This will assist you in maintaining or building your muscle, which will always keep your metabolism high. Muscle is the furnace that burns and shreds fat 24/7.

- **Use a fat-free diet that includes essential fats from supplements.** Your diet should be a balanced meal plan that revolves around carbohydrate for primary energy, and protein for muscle repair. This will fuel your body and encourage it to burn fat in between meals. A fat-free diet will create a fat deficit that will be replaced by your stored body fat. Essential fats must then be replaced manually, through supplementation.

- Always eat before a weight session at the gym. In order to get your very best performance and strength, your body must have food as energy. Take the opportunity to eat slightly more food in preparation for resistance exercise. This higher calorie intake will boost your metabolism, while you perform at your very best. The high-intensity training will assist you in burning those calories, and will continue to burn more energy afterward.

- Aim to get at least eight hours of sleep per night. Getting good sleep is critical to your success. Treat this time as sacred and prepare for it early. You need good sleep to be refreshed and energized for the following day. This will guarantee your long-term success on *Shred Body Fat*.

- Halve your workouts and double your intensity. This is one of the best pieces of advice that anyone can receive when doing resistance training to build muscle and strength. By focusing on your intensity, you are able to realize that less is more. Your success depends on the effort invested, not the amount of time invested. Quality over quantity.

A New Life

Once you reach your fat-loss goal, it is time to start adjusting your program to your life and the other things that you would like to be doing. Maintaining your new body is a lot easier, due to not having to create a deficit in calories. The weight that you lose will be gone permanently, because it is real fat-loss. Despite having reached your target, you can reintroduce foods, and not be as concerned about cutting every single gram of fat from your diet. By using the basic knowledge of daily fat needs (40 grams for women and 60 grams for men), weight control becomes a matter of transitioning from a fat-free diet to a low-fat diet.

You can also cut the number of days of cardio that you do in a week. This may be only 1 or 2 days. Your weight can be controlled by removing cardio entirely, and just monitoring your diet. Although this may sound appealing, there are many other health benefits to cardiovascular exercise, regardless of the body you have. Cutting down your cardio to make time for other things in your life, may be a wiser decision than cutting it out all together. Alternatively, you may choose to keep doing cardio 3-6 times a week, simply so you can live a more extravagant life and eat more of the foods that would normally be forbidden. Again, this may sound appealing, but moderation is always a smarter option.

In transitioning to a maintenance diet, I suggest increasing the level of good fats in your diet. Good fats in the form of omega-3 and omega-6 are essential fatty acids which benefit your body and brain performance, as well as lowering bad cholesterol (LDL). For muscle strength, I suggest that you continue to maintain resistant training with weights or machines, 2-3 times per week. Keeping the muscle that you have built during *Shred Body Fat* will be your biggest asset for maintaining your new body. Remember, muscle is the foundation of your metabolism.

Having a good balance between diet and exercise throughout the week will be a treat for your body. You should always aim to keep it strong and healthy. Combining the basic knowledge of macronutrients, fat intake, smart exercise and listening to your hunger signals, will ensure that you keep your new body. This is knowledge that will never leave you.

Belief

I'm going to leave this part short and sweet. The reason for this is that I have provided you with highly practical knowledge and all the tools necessary to reach your goal. Science proves that reaching your goal is inevitable if you apply what I have written in this book. Having said that, belief in yourself to achieve success in that area of your life is crucial. You need to have the belief that your application and discipline WILL pay off. I have presented you with the facts and a thorough understanding of how the body utilizes fat. This is what I believe to be 80% of the battle, of which I have already fought for you. Having the belief means erasing all the information that contradicts real scientific evidence, then starting from scratch. This will not let you down. Use it to fuel your determination. Once you start seeing the results that science and nature promises you, your belief will become unstoppable. Fat-loss will no longer be a mystery and you'll wonder how you never discovered these methods sooner.

Synergy

Synergy is the combined effect of many forces achieving a greater result than those individual forces done separately. In other terms, 1+1+1=10, not 3. It occurs in many things in life and can mean the difference between success and failure. In this case, synergy applies to the combination of nutrition, weight training and cardio. I have made each concept in this book simple enough to understand, but the challenge is to apply all the pieces together as a whole. The perfect way to shred body fat is through the combined application of all the principles in this book. As you master them, you will be forming permanent habits which will force your body to use fat as a source of energy. This will occur in a healthy and natural way. In turn, you will have the ability to sculpt and transform your body, without putting yourself in danger.

Use and treat this book as your key to achieving your goal, because it has everything that you will ever need. Refer back to the summary on page 158, to remind yourself of the most important parts in shredding fat. I have done my best to keep the information here as simple and practical as possible, in order to get the message across in the best way. I could have made this book another 300 pages longer, but it makes no sense to fill your mind will information that will only cloud your direct path to your goal. The principles of fat-loss are very simple and logical, so that's the way they should be expressed.

Try to have an open mind towards the ideas that I have presented to you regarding resistance and weight training. Some of them may be deemed as unorthodox by certain people, but decide for yourself after analyzing your own personal results. The most important thing is that you realize you do not need to spend countless hours in the gym to achieve strength gains. By shocking your muscle with an exercise that works best and a weight that challenges you, your body will be continually improving on its strength. This is a natural process, which will aid the natural process of shredding body fat, outlined in this book.

Remember, it doesn't matter who you are or what history you have of obesity and weight gain, you can shred as much fat from your body as you want. Science proves this beyond doubt and countless people before you have achieved it. There is absolutely no difference between you and those people who have succeeded in taking advantage of the way that all humans are programmed. It is simply a matter of whether you want it enough to apply the discipline of following the instructions in this book. The direct path to your desired body weight and fat-loss goal has been created. Now, all you have to do is walk down that path and do it.

Shred Body Fat